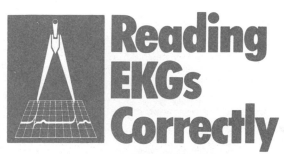

Reading EKGs Correctly

SECOND EDITION
NURSING84 BOOKS™
SPRINGHOUSE CORPORATION
SPRINGHOUSE, PENNSYLVANIA

NURSING84 BOOKS™

NEW NURSING SKILLBOOK™ SERIES
Giving Emergency Care Competently
Monitoring Fluid and Electrolytes Precisely
Assessing Vital Functions Accurately
Coping with Neurologic Problems Proficiently
Reading EKGs Correctly
Combatting Cardiovascular Diseases Skillfully
Nursing Critically Ill Patients Confidently
Dealing with Death and Dying

NURSING PHOTOBOOK™ SERIES
Providing Respiratory Care
Managing I.V. Therapy
Dealing with Emergencies
Giving Medications
Assessing Your Patients
Using Monitors
Providing Early Mobility
Giving Cardiac Care
Performing GI Procedures
Implementing Urologic Procedures
Controlling Infection
Ensuring Intensive Care
Coping with Neurologic Disorders
Caring for Surgical Patients
Working with Orthopedic Patients
Nursing Pediatric Patients
Helping Geriatric Patients
Attending Ob/Gyn Patients
Aiding Ambulatory Patients
Carrying Out Special Procedures

NURSE'S REFERENCE LIBRARY®
Diseases
Diagnostics
Drugs
Assessment
Procedures
Definitions
Practices
Emergencies

Nursing84 DRUG HANDBOOK™

NURSING NOW™
Shock
Hypertension
Drug Interactions
Cardiac Crises
Respiratory Emergencies

NURSE'S CLINICAL LIBRARY™
Cardiovascular Disorders
Respiratory Disorders
Endocrine Disorders
Neurologic Disorders
Renal and Urologic Disorders

Reading
EKGs
Correctly

NEW NURSING SKILLBOOK™
Series
PROGRAM DIRECTOR
Jean Robinson

CLINICAL DIRECTOR
Barbara McVan, RN

PROJECT MANAGER
Susan Rossi Williams

**Springhouse Corporation
Book Division**
CHAIRMAN
Eugene W. Jackson

PRESIDENT
Daniel L. Cheney

VICE-PRESIDENT AND
DIRECTOR
Timothy B. King

VICE-PRESIDENT, BOOK
OPERATIONS
Thomas A. Temple

VICE-PRESIDENT, PRODUCTION
AND PURCHASING
Bacil Guiley

RESEARCH DIRECTOR
Elizabeth O'Brien

Library of Congress Cataloging in
Publication Data

Main entry under title:

Reading EKGs correctly.
(New Nursing Skillbook series)
"Nursing84 books."
Rev. ed. of: Reading EKGs
correctly/by Margaret Van Meter
and Peter G. Lavine. ©1981.
Bibliography: p.
Includes index.
1. Electrocardiography—
Handbooks, manuals, etc.
2. Heart—Diseases—Diagnosis—
Handbooks, manuals, etc.
3. Cardiovascular disease
nursing—Handbooks, manuals,
etc. I. Van Meter, Margaret.
Reading EKGs correctly. II.
Springhouse Corporation. III.
Series: New nursing skillbook.
RC683.5.E5R385 1984
616.1'207547   83-20269
ISBN 0-916730-61-1

Staff for this edition:
BOOK EDITOR: Patricia R. Urosevich
CLINICAL EDITOR: Barbara McVan, RN
ASSISTANT EDITOR: Jo Lennon
DESIGNER: Kathaleen Motak Singel
COPY SUPERVISOR: David R. Moreau
COPY EDITORS: Susan L. Baumann, Diane M. Labus
EDITORIAL STAFF ASSISTANT: Ellen Johnson
ILLUSTRATORS: Robert Jackson, Mark Kudelka
ART PRODUCTION MANAGER: Robert Perry
ARTISTS: Diane Fox, Donald G. Knauss, Sandra Sanders, Craig Siman,
    Louise Stamper, Thom Staudenmayer, Scott M. Stephens
TYPOGRAPHY MANAGER: David C. Kosten
TYPOGRAPHY ASSISTANTS: Ethel Halle, Diane Paluba,
    Nancy Wirs
SENIOR PRODUCTION MANAGER: Deborah C. Meiris
PRODUCTION MANAGER: Wilbur D. Davidson
COVER ART: Ellis Chappell, ArtPeople

Clinical consultants for this edition:
Peter R. Kowey, MD, FACC, *Assistant Professor of Medicine; Director,
    Coronary Care Unit; Co-Director, Cardiovascular Research Laboratory,
    The Medical College of Pennsylvania, Philadelphia*
Kathleen R. Phillips, RN, CCRN, *Staff Development Instructor, Critical
    Care Units, Pennsylvania Hospital, Philadelphia*
Leslie K. Sampson, RN, CCRN, *Assistant Director of Continuing Nursing
    Education for Critical Care, The Medical College of Pennsylvania,
    Philadelphia*

Staff for first edition:
EDITOR: Patricia S. Chaney
TEXT EDITOR: Shirley Claypool
COPY EDITOR: Patricia A. Hamilton
PRODUCTION MANAGER: Bernard Haas
PRODUCTION ASSISTANTS: Grace Koontz, Laura Musmanno
DESIGNER: John C. Isely
ART DIRECTOR: Matie Patterson
ART ASSISTANT: Dale Swensson
PHOTOGRAPHER: Bill Baker

Clinical consultants for first edition:
Peter G. Lavine, MD, *Director, Coronary Care Division, Crozer-Chester
    Medical Center, Chester, Pa.*
Rose Pinneo, RN, MS, *Associate Professor of Nursing, University of
    Rochester, New York*
Margaret Van Meter, RN, *formerly Clinical Director, Nursing Magazine,
    Springhouse Corporation, Springhouse, Pa.*

Contents

Contributors

Peter R. Kowey is assistant professor of medicine, director of the coronary care unit, and co-director of the cardiovascular research laboratory of the Medical College of Pennsylvania in Philadelphia. A graduate of the University of Pennsylvania in Philadelphia, Dr. Kowey is a member of the American College of Cardiology, the North American Society of Pacing and Electrophysiology, the Cardiac Electrophysiology Society, and the American Federation for Clinical Research.

Peter G. Lavine is director of the coronary care unit of Crozer-Chester Medical Center in Chester, Pennsylvania. Before assuming that position, Dr. Lavine was director of the coronary care unit and assistant professor of medicine at Hahnemann Medical College and Hospital in Philadelphia. A graduate of Hahnemann Medical College, Dr. Lavine is a member of the American College of Physicians and the American College of Cardiology.

Suzanne A. Lavine is nearing completion of a BS degree in nursing at Widener University in Chester, Pennsylvania. After receiving a diploma from the Allentown (Pa.) Hospital School of Nursing, Ms. Lavine worked in the coronary care unit at Crozer-Chester Medical Center in Chester, Pennsylvania. She is a member of the American Association of Critical-Care Nurses and the American Nurses' Association.

Kathleen R. Phillips is staff development instructor for the critical care units at Pennsylvania Hospital in Philadelphia. She received her diploma from St. Joseph's Hospital School of Nursing in Reading, Pennsylvania.

Rose Pinneo is associate professor of nursing and clinician II at the University of Rochester in New York. She received her MS from the University of Pennsylvania, Philadelphia, and is a member of the American Association of Critical-Care Nurses.

Leslie K. Sampson is assistant director of continuing education for critical care, the Medical College of Pennsylvania in Philadelphia. A diploma graduate of the Philadelphia General Hospital School of Nursing, he's a BSN candidate at La Salle College in Philadelphia. He's also a member of the American Association of Critical-Care Nurses, the American Nurses' Association, and the Society of Critical Care Medicine.

Advisory Board

Foreword

Twenty years ago, few nurses knew how to analyze an electrocardiogram. And little wonder; most of them had never even seen one, much less had to evaluate one. Today, though, electrocardiographs, like thermometers, blood pressure cuffs, and stethoscopes, have become standard assessment tools. So, reading and interpreting EKG strips is significant not only for nurses in the cardiac care unit but also in doctors' offices, primary care divisions, emergency departments, and many nursing units in a hospital.

Although the cardiac clinical nurse specialist needs to assess and interpret the more complex strips, the vast number of nurses — from beginners to skilled cardiac nurse practitioners — need a clear, concise understanding of only the most common EKGs. And they want to be able to link this information to their basic knowledge of anatomy, chemistry, and physiology so the rationale behind electrocardiography can be meaningful to them. It is precisely to these goals that the editors of this fully updated Skillbook have dedicated their entire approach.

From beginning to end, they have designed explanations to reach the reader at her level of understanding. First, they give a basic account of the electrophysiology and conduction systems. Then, they outline the step-by-step method for analyzing any EKG for rate, rhythm, conduction, configuration, and location of waves. And finally, they explain all common dysrhythmias, each time focusing on the key questions: Where did it originate? What effect does it have on the heart? What treatment is necessary? What problems might the treatment create? What would happen to the patient if the problem were not corrected? And what are the implied special nursing considerations?

Interspersed throughout the second edition of *Reading EKGs Correctly* are interesting patient studies, so that theory is always linked with practice. At the end of each section and at the end of this Skillbook, the reader has numerous chances to test what she has learned.

Reading EKGs Correctly fills a definite need for a compact, interesting presentation of EKGs. By using this new and completely updated edition, the beginner should gain a rapid but thorough grasp of a sophisticated but relatively simple tool. Then, with continued study and practice, she can build on the basic skills she learns here to become truly proficient at EKG interpretation. With time at a premium, no practicing nurse can afford to pass up this practical manual and the enriching experience of painlessly learning the fundamentals of EKG interpretation.

LILLIAN S. BRUNNER, RN, MSN, ScD, FAAN
Consultant in Nursing
Presbyterian–University of
Pennsylvania Medical Center
Philadelphia

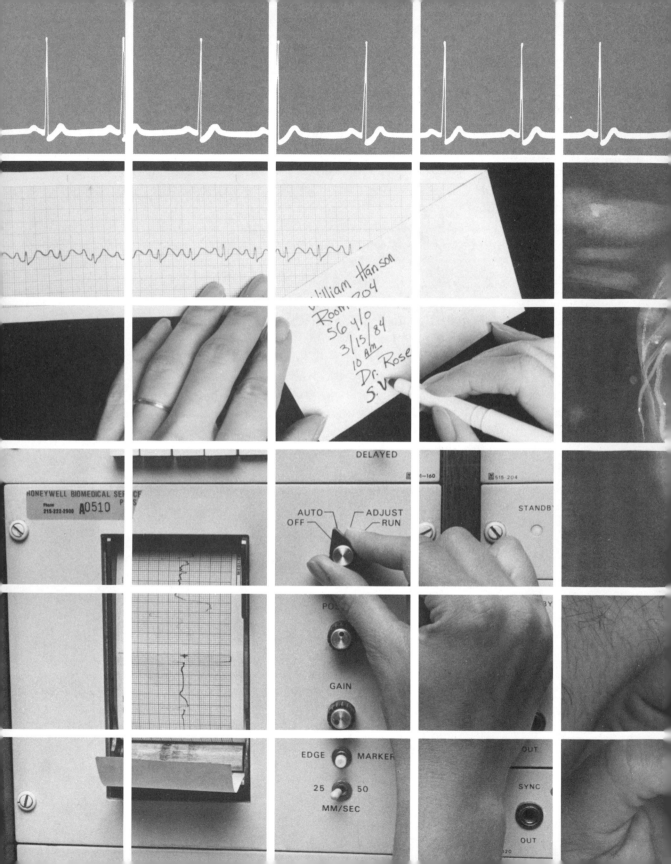

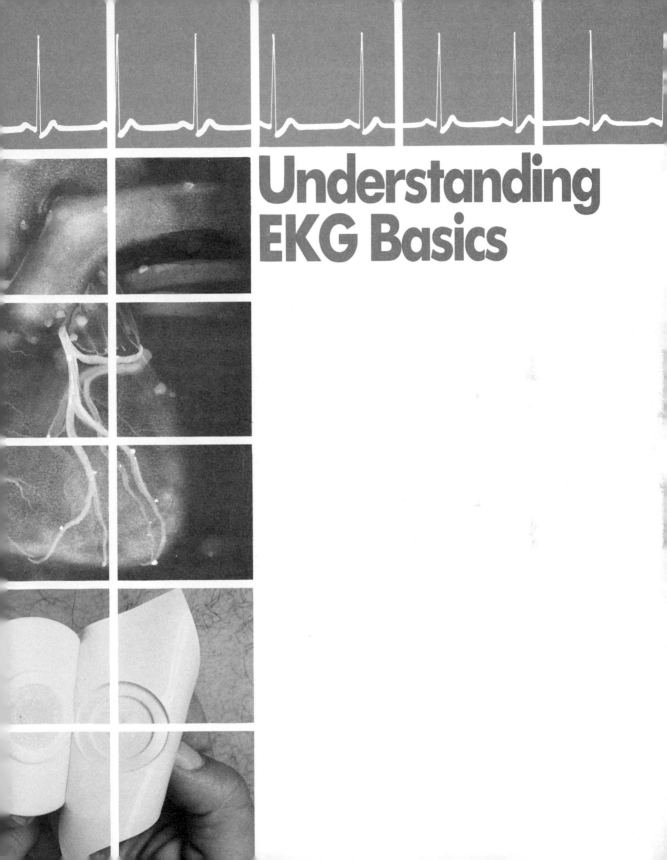

Understanding
EKG Basics

What occurs when a patient sustains a disturbance in any of the cardiac cycle's processes?

What five facts do you need to know to identify and understand a dysrhythmia?

If your patient's PR interval is slightly prolonged, where should you suspect a possible conduction delay?

What do tentlike T waves usually indicate?

If your patient has a premature QRS complex that's close to the T wave of the preceding beat, what type of ventricular abnormality would you suspect?

1

What does an EKG tell you about the heart?

Like so much modern electronic gadgetry, the electrocardiograph seems to possess an aura of mystery and magic. Even the terminology of EKG interpretation sounds like an occult code: QRS complexes, inverted P waves, RR intervals, and so forth.

As mysterious as it all sounds, however, the principles behind electrocardiography and EKG interpretation are fairly simple. In fact, with only a rudimentary understanding of the electrical systems of the heart and the EKG machine itself, you can make some general observations about a patient's EKG report.

Suppose, for example, you overheard a doctor explaining a patient's EKG as follows: "He's got good P waves and a slightly prolonged PR interval. But see how much his QRS has widened since last night!"

To evaluate the doctor's comments in a general sense, you need only to know the relationship between EKG waves and cardiac anatomy and to understand which parts of the heart the various EKG leads focus on. More concisely, you need to know something about the heart's electrophysiology and the standard 12-lead EKG system.

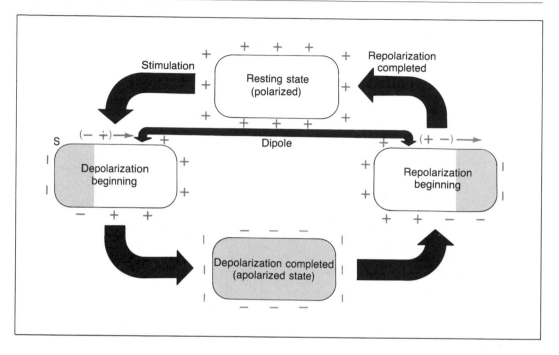

Cardiac depolarization-repolarization cycle
This diagram shows the depolarization-repolarization cycle as well as a simplified view of the electrical activity of the cardiac muscle. Since the architecture of the heart muscle cell and its membrane is very complex, the flow of electrical current through the heart is not simply a transfer of ions across a single membrane; it includes metabolic processes as well.

Electrophysiology of the heart

The many cells of the heart are arranged so that they act as one system or network. Two types of electrical processes, called *depolarization* and *repolarization* (illustrated above), are transmitted throughout this network. During depolarization, the cells are stimulated and the myocardium contracts; during repolarization, it relaxes. The entire process is called the cardiac cycle.

A disturbance in any of the processes of the cardiac cycle will cause a change in the electrical forces needed to maintain normal, rhythmic contractions and may produce a dysrhythmia. It could be anything from a minor disruption of rhythm to a major life-threatening dysrhythmia, depending on the degree of the disturbance.

During their resting stage, the cells of the myocardium are said to be *polarized* — that is, they have positive charges on the outside of each cell and an equal number of negative charges on the inside. Electrical stimulation makes the cell membrane permeable to the flow of ions, which is responsible for the flow of electrical current throughout the myocardium.

Sodium and potassium ions figure importantly in this elec-

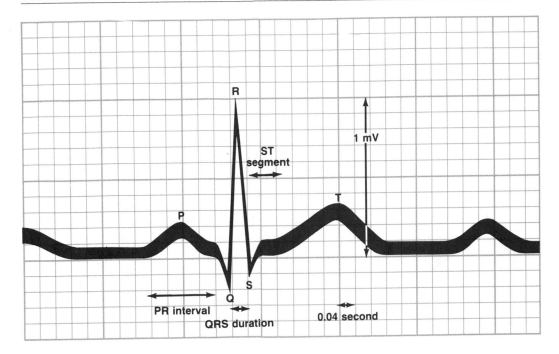

trical activity. In the resting cell, the potassium ion (K^+) concentration is 50 times greater inside the cell than outside while sodium ion concentration is greater outside the cell. Upon *depolarization*, the first current flow consists of sodium ions (Na^+) moving from outside to inside the cell until the outer surface becomes negatively charged and the membrane is fully depolarized. The flow of potassium ions from inside the cell to outside begins shortly after the sodium ions start to move in. When the potassium ion flow exceeds that of sodium ions, *repolarization* of the membrane begins, and the outer surface of the membrane again becomes positively charged.

To understand the electrical activity of the heart, think of the heart as consisting of two separate cell networks — one comprising the atria and the other the ventricles. Stimulation must spread through the muscle of both the atria and the ventricles before mechanical contraction can occur.

Each of these cell networks is considered separately on the electrocardiogram, which is simply a graphic recording of the electrical forces produced by the heart. In fact, all the waves of the EKG can be correlated with the level of electrical stimulation that precedes the heart's contraction and relaxation.

Minding your P's and Q's
Here you can see the EKG waves for one cardiac cycle. These waves have been arbitrarily labeled the P, QRS, and T waves.

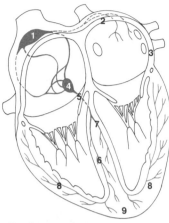

**Cardiac conduction:
Following the route**
The numbers on the heart above
trace the cardiac conduction
route. The key below tells you
which part of the heart's anatomy
corresponds with each number.
  1. Sinus node (SA node)
  2. Intraatrial tracts
  3. Atrial muscle fibers
  4. Atrioventricular node (AV
     node)
  5. Bundle of His
  6. Right bundle branch
  7. Superior and inferior divi-
     sions of left bundle branch
  8. Purkinje's fibers
  9. Ventricular muscle
  As you can see, the impulse
arrives first at the sinoatrial node,
works its way through the heart
chambers, and eventually
reaches the ventricular muscle.

The P wave reflects depolarization of the atria; the QRS complex reflects the depolarization of the ventricles; and the T wave reflects the repolarization of the ventricles. (The T wave corresponding to the repolarization of the atria is not visible in the figure on the previous page, because it is obscured by the QRS deflection.) The mass of the ventricles is much greater than that of the atria, so the QRS and T waves are much larger than the P wave.

Occasionally, another wave will appear after the T wave. Called the U wave, it usually shows up on the EKGs of patients who have low serum potassium levels. The wave can usually be eliminated by giving a potassium supplement. (In recent laboratory studies, U waves have been produced in animals during the repolarization stages of the Purkinje's fibers.)

Cardiac conduction

Stimulation of the heart originates in the sympathetic and parasympathetic branches of the autonomic nervous system. The impulse travels first to the sinoatrial (SA) node, located in the posterior wall of the right atrium near the orifice of the superior vena cava (see illustration at left). The SA node is the main cardiac pacemaker, from which wavelike impulses are sent through the atria, stimulating first the right and then the left atrium.

As soon as the atria have been stimulated, the impulse slows as it passes through the atrioventricular (AV) node. This node is located near the intraventricular septum in the inferior wall of the right atrium and near the tricuspid valve.

Slowing of the impulse at the AV node allows the ventricles, which are resting (diastole), to fill with blood from the atria. The wave of excitation (stimulation) then spreads to the bundle of His, the left and right bundle branches, and the Purkinje's fibers, which terminate in the ventricles. Stimulation of the muscle of the ventricle begins in the intraventricular septum and moves downward, causing ventricular depolarization and contraction. Mechanically, the ventricles empty into the pulmonary (or lesser) circulation and the systemic (or greater) circulation.

The 12-lead EKG system

The basic electrocardiograph has electrodes that are attached to the arms and legs plus a floating electrode for the precordial,

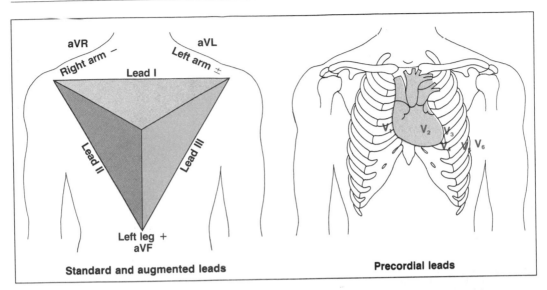

Standard and augmented leads

Precordial leads

or chest, leads. Most hospitals use a standard 12-lead system that records activity from the frontal and horizontal planes of the body.

The *standard limb leads,* known as leads I, II, and III, are called bipolar leads, because each of them has two electrodes that record simultaneously the electrical forces of the heart flowing toward two extremities. That is, lead I records electrical activity between the right arm and left arm; lead II records activity between the right arm and left leg; and lead III records activity between the left leg and left arm.

The right arm is always considered to be the negative pole, while the left leg is always the positive pole. The left arm can be either positive or negative, depending on the lead — in lead I, it is positive; in lead III, it is negative.

When current flows toward the positive pole, the deflections of the EKG wave will be upright (positive). When current flows toward the negative pole, the deflections will be inverted (negative). In lead II the flow of the current is from the negative to the positive, so the deflections on the normal EKG will be upright.

The next three leads are known as *augmented leads,* so-called because they are designed to increase the amplitude of the deflections by 50% over those recorded by the standard limb leads (see above left). Augmented leads are unipolar; they record frontal plane activity, as the limb leads do. Be-

Getting into position
During an EKG, properly placed electrodes allow you to record the heart's electrical potential from 12 views. The illustration at left represents the standard limb leads and the unipolar augmented leads with their corresponding electrical charge.

The illustration at right shows the six unipolar precordial leads, or chest leads (V_1 through V_6). Remember to avoid placing these electrodes over the ribs.

The following are the proper positions for chest leads:

V_1 — fourth intercostal space at right border of sternum

V_2 — fourth intercostal space at left border of sternum

V_3 — halfway between V_2 and V_4

V_4 — fifth intercostal space at midclavicular line

V_5 — anterior axillary line (halfway between V_4 and V_6)

V_6 — midaxillary line, level with V_4.

Getting a readout

These tracings are from a normal 12-lead EKG. If you keep in mind that each lead gives a picture of a different anatomic part of the heart, you can pinpoint areas of damage more easily.

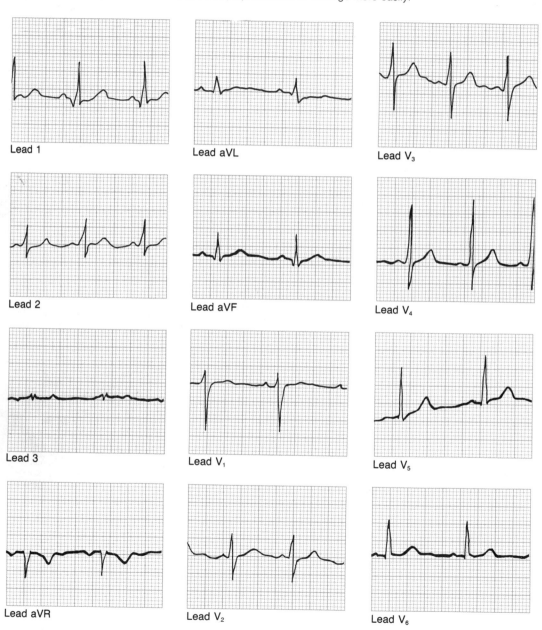

Lead 1

Lead aVL

Lead V₃

Lead 2

Lead aVF

Lead V₄

Lead 3

Lead V₁

Lead V₅

Lead aVR

Lead V₂

Lead V₆

cause they record activity from the right and left shoulders and left leg, they are identified as aVR (augmented right), aVL (augmented left), and aVF (augmented foot). By studying all six leads, you will get more information than from the three standard leads alone.

The remaining six leads of the 12-lead system are the unipolar *precordial leads,* or chest leads (see illustration top right on page 17). They are designated by the letter "V" and a number that represents the position of the electrode on the chest wall, or precordium. These positions are: V_1 — fourth intercostal space, right sternal border; V_2 — fourth intercostal space, left sternal border; V_3 — midway between V_2 and V_4, on a line joining these two locations; V_4 — fifth intercostal space in midclavicular line; V_5 — fifth intercostal space in anterior axillary line; and V_6 — fifth intercostal space in midaxillary line.

The placement of the precordial leads in relation to the ventricles gives a good picture of the electrical activity within the ventricles themselves. Leads V_1 and V_2 represent the right ventricle (and also the right atrium), while leads V_3 through V_6 represent the larger left ventricle. Therefore, these six leads will increase the amplitude of the R wave and decrease the amplitude of the S wave from V_1 to V_6 respectively.

Applying your knowledge

Now, go back to the doctor's explanation of one patient's EKG in the beginning of this chapter. Are you ready to evaluate it?

The doctor's first statement, that the P waves are normal, should tell you that the patient's atria seem to be functioning normally. His second statement, that the PR interval is slightly prolonged, should lead you to suspect a possible delay in the atrioventricular conduction time (AV node). And his statement that the QRS complex is becoming wider should lead you to suspect some cardiac abnormality in the ventricles or their conduction systems. Remember, these are only educated guesses that you must now prove or disprove.

To decide what is causing abnormalities in the EKG, you must closely examine the patient's EKG. Precisely measure the various waves and intervals, and know the patient's history and current treatment. Only then can you determine if the patient has a cardiac problem, where it is, what it is, and what to do about it.

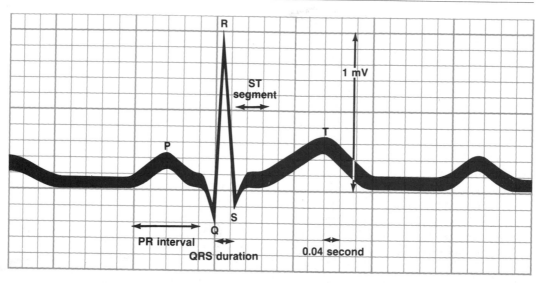

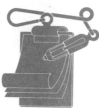

As you study this tracing, remember these important points:
1. The P wave indicates SA node function, which is produced by atrial depolarization. This wave is best seen in leads II and V_1, where it is normally upright.
2. The PR interval indicates atrioventricular conduction time. The interval is measured from the onset of the P wave to the beginning of the QRS complex. Normal PR interval: 0.12 to 0.20 second; a short PR interval indicates that the impulse originates in an area other than the SA node; and a long PR interval indicates that the impulse is delayed as it passes through the AV node.
3. The Q wave is the first negative (inverted) deflection following the P wave and the PR interval.
4. The R wave is the first positive (upright) deflection after the Q wave. (If no Q waves are visible, the R wave is the first upright deflection after the PR interval.)
5. The S wave is the first negative deflection following the R wave.
6. The ST segment is an isoelectric (flat) line having no voltage, from the end of the S wave to the beginning of the T wave.
7. The T wave indicates repolarization of the ventricles; follows the S wave and the ST segment.
8. The QRS duration indicates the time in which ventricular depolarization occurs. Normal duration: 0.06 to 0.10 second.

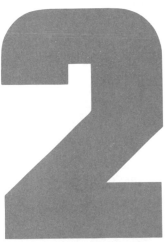

Forging a format for interpretation

Imagine you're a med-surg nurse who's been pulled to the ICU. Shortly after 4 a.m. you get a call that a patient is being admitted to your unit.

The patient, you're told, has suffered an apparent myocardial infarction, but because the CCU has no beds available, he'll spend the rest of the night in the ICU. He has typical symptoms: severe, crushing chest pains radiating down his left arm — pain that has persisted despite morphine administered by his family doctor before admission. His pulse is 44 and regular (sinus bradycardia); his blood pressure, 90/70. His skin feels cold and clammy; he's perspiring profusely.

On admission the doctor administers oxygen, starts an I.V. of dextrose 5% in water, and gives atropine, 0.5 mg I.V. He orders lab studies: arterial blood gases, electrolytes, cardiac enzymes, CBC, and prothrombin time. He also orders continuous monitoring of the patient's heart. While the doctor is writing his orders, you apply electrodes to the patient's chest and attach the lead wires to a cardiac monitor.

Once the doctor has left, you check his orders: "Monitor continuously. Notify me of any changes in rate, rhythm, or conduction; or of any signs of myocardial irritability, such as

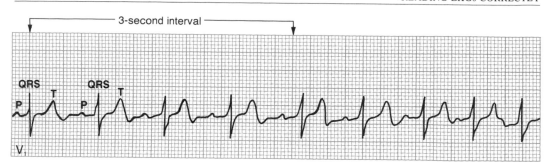

Exercising your skills

1. Rate
    (a) Atrial _____
    (b) Ventricular _____

2. Rhythm
    (a) Atrial _____
    (b) Ventricular _____

3. Conduction
    (a) PR interval _____
    (b) QRS duration _____

4. Configuration and location
    (a) P wave _____
    (b) QRS complex _____
    (c) ST segment _____
    (d) T wave _____

5. Summary _____
_____
_____
_____

(Answers on page 26)

PVCs; or signs of reduced cardiac output or congestive heart failure. Give atropine, 0.5 mg I.V., for a rate of 50 or below.''

Understanding the doctor's orders
Do you know what the doctor hoped to achieve by administering atropine and how to use the monitor to assess the effect of the drug? How confident do you feel about your ability to detect changes in your patient's cardiac rhythm? What signs would alert you to deteriorating cardiac output or congestive heart failure?

    To answer the first question we posed, the doctor gave atropine to speed the patient's sinus rate and, in turn, improve his cardiac output and coronary perfusion. By 6:30 a.m., when the EKG was taken, the atropine had produced the intended effect: the patient's pulse remained above 50. The improvement in the patient's heart action was apparent from the EKG (as we shall see); of course, it was also clinically apparent. Indeed, if the atropine had not been effective — if the patient's cardiac output had not improved — he would have felt lightheaded, developed syncope, and even had convulsive seizures. If the bradycardia had persisted, eventually he would have developed signs of congestive heart failure.

Interpreting an EKG
Let's begin with a very basic, step-by-step analysis of the rhythm strip (shown above) as a practical way of presenting the basic format you can apply when reading any strip. (Although there are other methods you can use to interpret a rhythm strip, we've found the following method to be the easiest to use.)

    As you read through the following procedure, study the rhythm strip and then write your interpretations in the blank spaces provided beneath it. In this way, you'll be developing the information you need in order to properly care for your patient.

● *Rate*. When we talk about heart rate, we generally mean the ventricular rate, which you can easily feel in a pulse. But to accurately assess an EKG tracing, you'll need to know both the atrial and ventricular rates. First, find the atrial rate.

Since the P wave indicates sinus (or sinoatrial) activity, you must first identify the P wave in the rhythm strip (the waves have been labeled for your convenience). Now find two consecutive P waves. Count the number of small squares between the two P waves — you may use either the apex of the wave or the initial upstroke of the wave.

Each small square is equal to 0.04 second; thus, 1,500 small squares equal 1 minute ($0.04 \times 1,500 = 60$ seconds = 1 minute). So, you divide 1,500 by the number of squares you counted between the P waves. This will give you the atrial rate — the number of atrial contractions/minute. Write your answer on line 1(a) beneath the rhythm strip.

Now locate the QRS complexes in the rhythm strip. (QRS is more easily identified because it is usually the tallest of the waves on the tracing. Normally, the QRS complex should be 10 small squares high, or 1 mV.) Again, count the number of small squares between the R waves of two consecutive QRS complexes. Divide 1,500 by the number of small squares to find the ventricular rate — the number of ventricular contractions/minute. (If the patient's rhythm is *regular*, you may make your calculations using the calibration table on page 141.) Then write your answer on line 1(b).

(*Note:* If the rhythm is irregular, counting the squares in a *single* RR interval will give you an approximate rather than a precise rate, which you would get with a perfectly regular rhythm.)

● *Rhythm*. To determine whether your patient's heart rhythm is regular or irregular, you will again need to know the atrial and ventricular activity. Find the atrial rhythm first, referring to the two consecutive P waves. For this, you'll need either calipers, or a piece of paper with a straight edge and a pencil with a sharp point (see photographs on next page).

If you're using the paper-and-pencil method, place the straight edge of your paper along the baseline of the rhythm strip. Then, move the paper up slightly so that the straight

Quick count
A faster way to determine atrial rate is to count the P waves in a 3-second strip and multiply this number by 20. (In a 6-second strip, count the P waves and multiply by 10.)

You determine the ventricular rate in the same way — just count the R waves instead of the P waves.

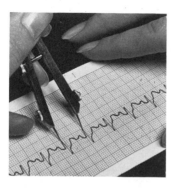

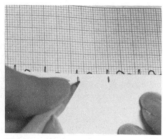

Measure the tracing with calipers...or with a piece of paper.

edge is near the top peak of the P waves. With your pencil, make a dot on the paper at each of two consecutive P waves (bottom photograph); this is the PP interval. Now, move the paper across the strip from left to right, lining up the two dots with each consecutive P wave. If the distance between all of the P waves is the same, the atrial rhythm is regular; if the distance varies, the rhythm is irregular. Write your answer on line 2(a) on page 22.

Then, using the same method, measure the distance between the R waves of consecutive QRS complexes (the RR interval) to determine whether the ventricular rhythm is regular or irregular. Record your answer on line 2(b). Note, also, whether the rhythm is only slightly irregular or markedly irregular.

● *Conduction.* Conduction is the time it takes for the impulse originating at the SA node to stimulate ventricular contraction.

Conduction time is found by measuring the PR interval and the QRS duration. To measure the PR interval, count the number of small squares from the beginning of the P wave to the beginning of the R wave. Multiply this number by 0.04 second. This tells you how long it has taken the electrical impulse to travel from the SA node through the atria and through the AV node to the bundle of His in the ventricles. Write your answer on line 3(a).

To determine the QRS duration, count the number of small squares from the beginning of the Q wave to the beginning of the ST segment and multiply by 0.04 second. However, when the Q wave is absent (as in the tracing on page 22) you'll measure the duration starting with the R wave. This tells you how long it takes for the electrical impulse to be conducted through the ventricle. Write this answer on line 3(b).

● *Configuration and location.* The configuration and location of the waves on a rhythm strip also tell you something about the extent and location of myocardial damage or the source of cardiac impulses.

First, look carefully at all of the P waves. Study their configuration. Are they similar in shape and size? If not, it might mean irritability in the atrial tissue or damage near the SA node. Of course, certain drugs may also cause this effect. Do all of the P waves point in the same direction — are all upright, all inverted, or all diphasic (consisting of both upright and inverted segments)? Is this configuration normal for the lead being recorded?

Next, examine the location of the P waves. Does a P wave precede each QRS complex? Are they present at all? Are they closer to the T wave in some beats? Write your answers on line 4(a).

Next, look at the QRS complexes. Ask yourself the same questions you asked about the P waves: What are their shape, size, and direction; what is their location in relation to the T waves? Also, look at their relation to the P waves.

A premature QRS complex that is close to the T wave of the preceding beat spells danger for the patient because it means that the ventricles, irritated by ectopic stimulation, are contracting prematurely. The closer this ectopic beat is to the T wave (which represents the period of ventricular relaxation), the greater the chances of severe ventricular dysrhythmia.

Do the QRS complexes occur in groups or clusters — that is, do two or more QRS complexes appear in rapid succession? Record your findings on line 4(b).

Now look at the ST segment. (An ST segment abnormality provides one of the earliest clues in diagnosing myocardial infarction.) Normally, this is a flat (isoelectric) line that is measured from the end of the S wave (of the QRS complex) to the beginning of the T wave. To determine if the ST segment is elevated or depressed, place the straight edge of the paper along the baseline of the rhythm strip. Look at the ST segment: Is it on a straight line with the PR interval? Does it extend above the baseline (elevated)? Or, is it below the baseline (depressed)? Record your observations on line 4(c).

Finally, look at the T waves. Evaluate the size and shape of each one in comparison with the other T waves. All T waves should be the same size and shape throughout the tracing. Also, they should point in the same direction as the QRS complexes and should follow them. Record your observations on line 4(d).

The QT interval is also measured because it reflects such influences as drugs. To measure this interval, count the small squares from the beginning of the QRS complex to the end of the T wave, and multiply this number by 0.04 second. The normal interval ranges from 0.32 to 0.42 second, depending on the ventricular rate.

Now go back over the findings you've recorded and try to group them so you can understand them. If you find an area in which an irregularity appears, try to figure out whether there

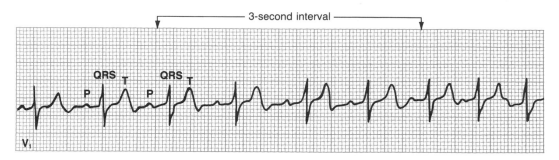

— 3-second interval —

QRS   T   QRS   T

P   P

V₁

is a pattern to the irregularity or whether it is confined to just one place. For example, if the RR interval changes with each cycle, you'll know that the ventricular rhythm is grossly irregular. The same is true of the PP interval.

Now, record your summary on line 5 and compare your answers with those at left.

Interpreting your findings

Before your shift ends, the doctor calls to check on the patient's condition. You report that he is resting quietly, without apparent pain. Further, the monitor shows his heart rate (ventricular rate) is now 84 beats/minute, with some irregularity in the atrial and ventricular rhythms. The QRS complex has not changed in size, shape, or direction, but some of the P waves have now become inverted and the RR interval has shortened. The PR interval and QRS duration are within normal limits.

Because of the EKG changes, the doctor decides to come to the unit and review the EKG strip with you. These are his findings:

"The presence of P waves and a normal PR interval preceding the QRS complex, together with a heart rate between 60 and 100, meet the criteria for normal sinus rhythm. (Sinus rhythms are discussed in the next chapter.) When the P wave changed direction, the RR interval shortened; these irregularities are premature beats, which can be assumed to originate above the ventricles in the nodal tissue because the QRS did not change.

"Elevation of the ST segment means ischemia or injury compatible with the admission diagnosis of myocardial infarction.

"Tentlike T waves are often seen with elevated serum potassium, so we'll have to check the serum electrolyte values immediately.

"The supraventricular or AV junctional premature beats mean that some atrial irritability is also present. We'll now have to watch the patient for other dysrhythmias, such as atrial fibrillation, paroxysmal atrial tachycardia, atrial flutter, and possibly junctional tachycardia."

Identifying dysrhythmias

What does this evaluation mean for this particular patient? How can you recognize the various dysrhythmias? As you work through the following chapters, the answers to those questions should become clear. But before we delve into specifics, let's take a look at dysrhythmias in general — what they are and what they mean for you and your patient.

Simply stated, a dysrhythmia is a disturbance in the cardiac rate or rhythm, or in the conduction of impulses through the heart. Dysrhythmias may be caused by several conditions: hypoxia, drug effects, electrolyte imbalance, and myocardial damage, to name a few.

The disturbance may be single, such as a rapid heart rate; or it may be multiple, such as rapid atrial rate, AV or intraventricular conduction delay, and premature ventricular contractions (PVCs). Combinations of dysrhythmias are possible and occur often.

The significance of each dysrhythmia depends on the patient's cardiac status and his systemic reaction to the disturbance. Some patients may be discharged even with a major dysrhythmia, such as PVCs; others with relatively minor dysrhythmias may be kept in the ICU.

Whatever the dysrhythmia, you'll need to know certain facts to identify and understand it:

1. Where did the dysrhythmia originate?

2. What's happening to the heart's conduction system?

3. What treatment would be needed to correct the dysrhythmia, and what problems might that treatment create?

4. What would happen to the patient if the dysrhythmia were not treated?

5. What special nursing considerations are implied by this dysrhythmia?

1. *Where did the dysrhythmia originate?* Normally, all cardiac impulses originate in the SA node, then progress through

the atria, the AV node, and the ventricular conduction fibers to the ventricles without any abnormal interference. Normally the presence of upright P waves on the EKG strip means the impulse began in the SA node.

Hidden or absent P waves mean that the impulse came from the AV node or even the ventricles. In this case, you should examine the QRS complex: Is it wide or normal? A wide QRS suggests the stimulus originated in the ventricles. A 12-lead EKG can best answer these questions, but a lead II or V_1 is a good, quick starting point for assessment.

2. *What's happening to the heart's conduction system?* Is the heart beating too fast (faster than 100 beats/minute)? Or, is it beating too slowly (slower than 60 beats/minute)? Is the beat irregular? Is it chaotically irregular, or is there some pattern to the irregularity? Is the atrial rate faster or slower than the ventricular rate? If it is faster, can you divide the atrial rate by the ventricular rate to yield a whole number (4:1, 3:1, or 2:1)? If you do not get a whole number something (AV block, for instance) is interfering with impulses passing through the AV node.

Remember, conduction normally slows somewhat at the AV node and the ventricular conduction bundles to allow the ventricles to fill with blood, but the delay should be brief (normal PR interval).

3. *What treatment would be needed to correct the dysrhythmia, and what problems might the treatment create?* Until recently, the mainstay of dysrhythmia treatment has been drug therapy — notably digitalis, propranolol (Inderal), and quinidine. Although most patients can tolerate aggressive drug therapy, some react unfavorably to certain drugs, presenting obstacles to dysrhythmia control. For example, a patient receiving digitalis for atrial fibrillation could develop a more serious dysrhythmia (PVC) due to digitalis toxicity or slow ventricular rates.

Other patients will fail to respond to aggressive therapy with digitalis or propranolol and may require a pacemaker or countershock to correct the dysrhythmia. However, the presence of high digitalis levels in a patient's blood increases the chances of cardiac arrest or dangerous dysrhythmias from the countershock.

Currently, temporary pacemakers are being used much more frequently to treat dysrhythmias because they are both effective and safe if properly positioned, and if supervised by an experienced and knowledgeable nursing and medical staff.

4. *What would happen to the patient if the dysrhythmia were not treated?* Sometimes nothing. If cardiac output and tissue perfusion are not impaired, the patient may require no treatment even though the dysrhythmia persists.

On the other hand, dysrhythmias that impair cardiac output usually must be treated. Rates that are too fast, rates that are too slow, or very irregular rhythms greatly reduce cardiac output. If the left ventricle fails to contract forcefully, blood backs up into the atria and, subsequently, into the pulmonary vasculature. The end result will be congestive heart failure.

A dysrhythmia can also create other problems. Diminished cardiac output means diminished perfusion of the brain, kidneys, liver, and myocardium, which in turn causes changes in sensorium and patient behavior, an enlarged and tender liver, and, in time, even jaundiced skin. Eventually, the kidneys shut down as the body attempts to conserve its sodium-water balance; the lungs become unable to handle the gas exchanges at the alveolar levels because of the excess fluid backup; and tissue hypoxia from poor coronary circulation to the myocardium will cause the patient to develop additional, more serious dysrhythmias.

The dysrhythmias most important to the patient are those that cause poor perfusion. They are considered dangerous and always require some type of treatment. Sometimes they can be reversed, sometimes not. Whether or not they respond to treatment depends on the condition of the heart muscle, especially the left ventricle. If there is extensive muscle damage, the prognosis is usually very poor.

5. *What special nursing considerations are implied?* You should carefully observe both the patient and his monitor. Even if you're inexperienced in dysrhythmia identification, you can notice whether the rate or rhythm changes. You can and certainly should always evaluate your patient clinically. How does he look? This is your most important clue to his condition. Especially observe his color, behavior, vital signs, and fluid intake and output. Finally, always keep in mind your basic responsibilities: try to give him a feeling of confidence in you and your judgment, try to anticipate his needs, and know when to call the doctor and what he might ask for when he treats the patient.

Systematic practice

With these basic facts in mind, you can begin interpreting the EKG strips in the following chapters. As you do, always keep in mind that the key to learning to interpret a rhythm strip is to keep to *one* fact-finding format. Do not omit any steps. Know *what* you are looking for and *why* you are looking for it. And practice the technique with the strips provided in this book and those recorded in your hospital. If you can find someone to practice with, so much the better.

Until you're sure of yourself, write down all of your findings. Then go back and interpret each one as it relates to the others.

If you work in an area that doesn't have continuous monitoring equipment, you can still practice every day by reading the patients' charts and analyzing the EKGs in them. If you know an EKG technician, ask her to save extra strips for you or to run some rhythm strips on the patients in your unit. Keep a notebook for yourself with the strips and your interpretations. Then compare how your results match up with the cardiologist's when his interpretation is placed in the chart.

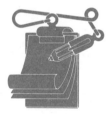

Remember these important points when interpreting an EKG:
1. Be alert for signs of poor cardiac output, for example, light-headedness, syncope, and convulsions.
2. Determine ventricular heart rate by counting the number of small squares between the R waves of two consecutive QRS complexes. Then, divide 1,500 by the number of small squares.
3. Irregularly sized and shaped P waves may indicate atrial tissue irritability or damage near the SA node.
4. Consider an ST segment abnormality an early clue to myocardial infarction.
5. Remember that atropine improves cardiac output and coronary perfusion by increasing the sinus rate.

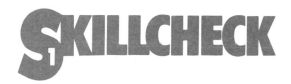

SKILLCHECK

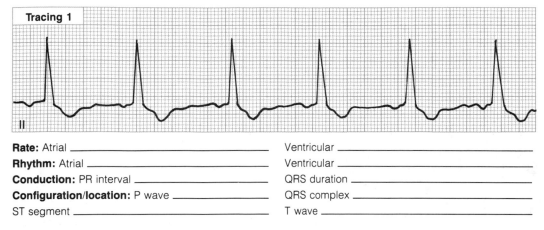

Tracing 1

II

Rate: Atrial _____ Ventricular _____

Rhythm: Atrial _____ Ventricular _____

Conduction: PR interval _____ QRS duration _____

Configuration/location: P wave _____ QRS complex _____

ST segment _____ T wave _____

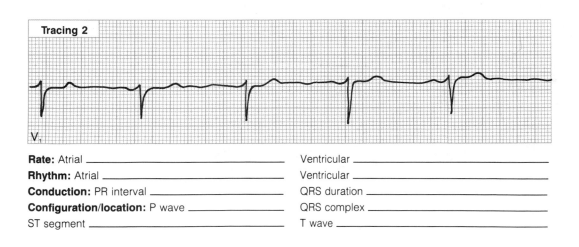

Tracing 2

V₁

Rate: Atrial _____ Ventricular _____

Rhythm: Atrial _____ Ventricular _____

Conduction: PR interval _____ QRS duration _____

Configuration/location: P wave _____ QRS complex _____

ST segment _____ T wave _____

(Answers on page 139)

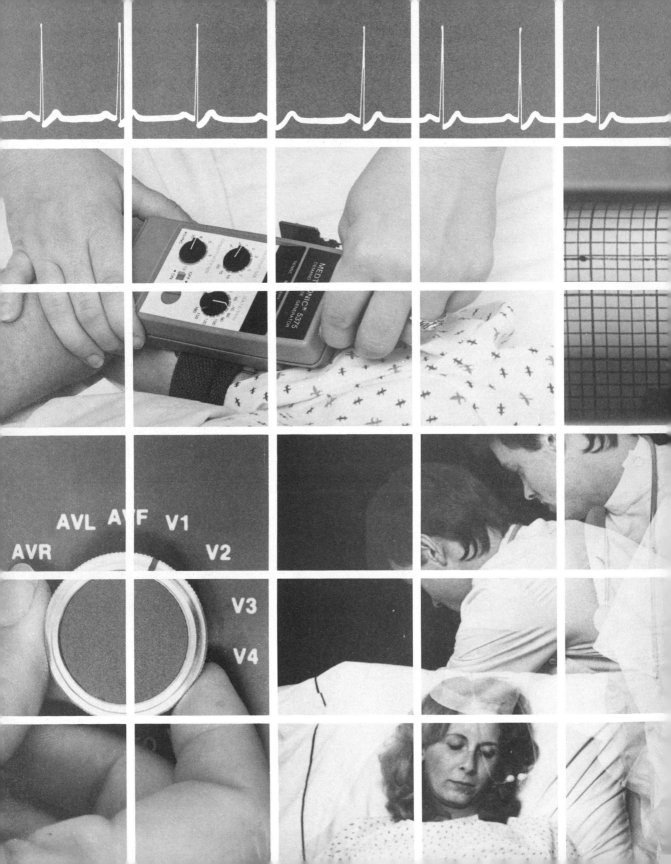

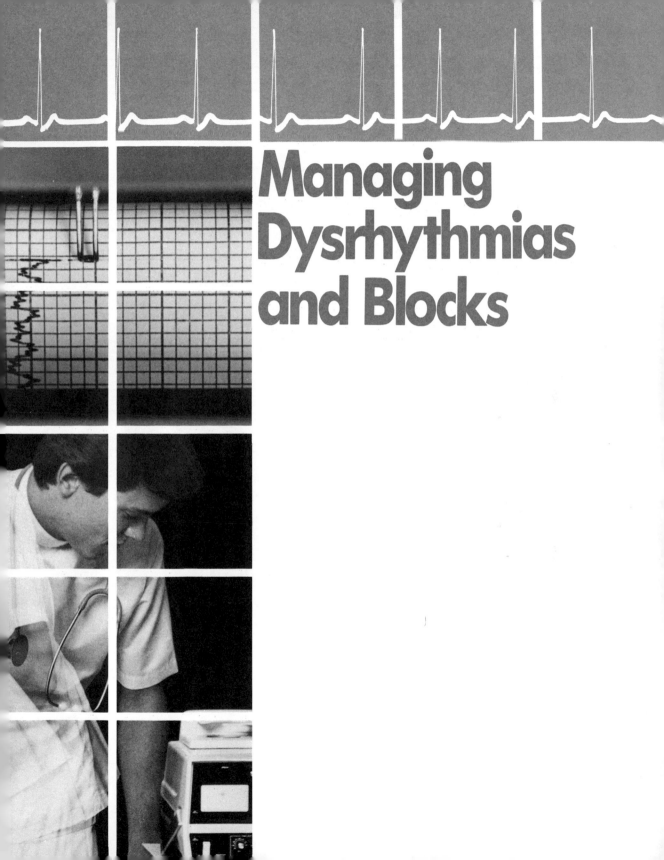

Managing Dysrhythmias and Blocks

What dysrhythmia would you expect to find in an athletic patient who has a sinus rate below 60 beats/minute?

Why would you avoid performing cardioversion on a patient with mitral stenosis and atrial fibrillation?

What ventricular contraction rate would you look for in a patient with a junctional dysrhythmia caused by digitalis toxicity?

If your patient with an anterior wall myocardial infarction develops a complete AV block, what symptoms would you expect to find?

If your patient has PVCs, what two signs will you find on his rhythm strip?

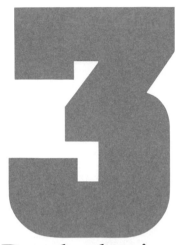

Dysrhythmias
of the SA node:
Serious or insignificant?

A good place to begin any discussion of specific dysrhythmias is with the most common — those of the SA node. These are generally considered the least dangerous of all dysrhythmias. For that reason, many nurses hold the mistaken idea that they are never serious. True, in 99 cases out of 100, they may not be. But in that 100th case, they may indeed be serious, even fatal.

Consider, for example, the case of John S., a laborer who had moderate chest pain for several days and was admitted to the CCU for observation and tests. Whenever the nurse glanced at John's EKG, she saw a normal P wave preceding a normal QRS complex, an apparently consistent RR interval, and an apparently consistent PP interval. So, she assumed that John had a normal sinus rhythm. She was wrong. Five hours after he was admitted, John developed an atrial tachycardia that progressed into congestive heart failure. What had gone wrong? With just casual glances at the monitor, and without analyzing the strip, the nurse had failed to detect the minute variations in the PP intervals, which may indicate sinus arrhythmias and can precede dangerous atrial dysrhythmias.

Fortunately, John survived. But his experience illustrates

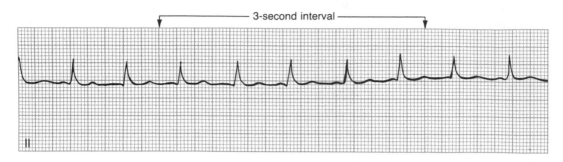

3-second interval

II

Normal sinus rhythm
EKG criteria:
- P wave is normal (of sinus node origin) and upright in lead II.
- P wave precedes each QRS complex.
- PR intervals are normal (0.12 to 0.2 second) and constant.
- RR intervals are constant.
- Heart rate falls between 60 and 100 beats/minute.

Treatment
- None is required.

just how serious dysrhythmias of the SA node can be. It also underlines the first important lesson about EKG interpretation: *You must never take anything for granted.* Just because a patient's EKG appears normal, as John's did, you can't assume that it is without a detailed analysis. Just because dysrhythmias of the SA node are common, you can't assume that they are inconsequential. And just because an EKG is a valuable diagnostic tool, you can't assume that it will give you all the answers about a patient's condition. Only by questioning, analyzing, and critically evaluating EKGs and then coupling those findings with information on the patient's medical history, lab tests, and diagnosis can you use the EKG as a valuable assessment tool.

With that in mind, let's examine those common — but not necessarily inconsequential — dysrhythmias of the SA node.

Recognizing the norm
Before you can learn to identify any abnormal rhythm, you naturally must learn to recognize the standard against which they are measured — normal sinus rhythm. What is a sinus rhythm? Basically, it is a rhythm that originates in the SA node, the heart's pacemaker and the origin of all normal heartbeats. On an electrocardiogram, sinus rhythms are characterized by the presence of a P wave of normal contour and a normal PR interval preceding each QRS complex.

Since the SA node is "programmed" to comfortably initiate 60 to 100 beats/minute, a normal sinus rhythm for an adult falls within that range. But normal sinus rates differ at different ages. At birth, rates of 110 to 150 beats/minute are common. But by age 6, the rates have slowed down to approximately those of adults.

In a normal sinus rhythm (shown above), the heart rate falls

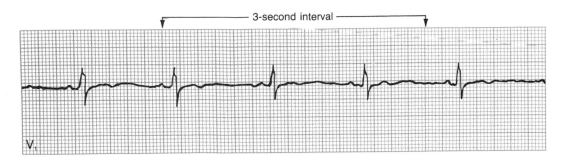

3-second interval

V₁

between 60 and 100 beats/minute. The other hallmarks of a normal sinus rhythm include a P wave, always preceding a QRS complex, and constant or fixed PR, PP, and RR intervals. Any deviation from these patterns signifies a dysrhythmia. If the dysrhythmia originates in the SA node, it will be one of the following.

• *Sinus bradycardia.* In the dysrhythmia shown above, the sinus rate is below 60 beats/minute, but all impulses still come from the SA node. Sinus bradycardia may be found in persons whose health is considered normal — especially athletes who are well conditioned. But it may also be one sign of underlying heart disease, such as myocardial infarction.

• *Sinus tachycardia.* In this dysrhythmia (see EKG strip on next page) the heart rate is from 100 to 160 beats/minute. Sinus tachycardia may be found in persons whose health is normal. It may be related to anxiety or strenuous exercise. Patients who don't have heart disease may experience sinus tachycardia with a fever or with hyperthyroidism. Or, this dysrhythmia can be an early manifestation of congestive heart failure or shock.

Rapid rates — more than 160 beats/minute — are considered to originate in an ectopic focus other than the SA node. For many patients whose rate is above 140, P waves will not be visible on the rhythm strip. For these patients, a 12-lead EKG should be taken to determine the exact location of the dysrhythmia (atrial, juctional, or ventricular).

• *Sinus arrhythmia.* A normal variation in sinus rhythm, when the rhythm has slight irregularities, is called sinus arrhythmia (see top EKG strip on page 39). Often, a rhythm strip will appear to be normal; only by measuring each PP or RR interval will you find a slight variation of the atrial rhythm.

The most common type of sinus arrhythmia is found in

Sinus bradycardia
EKG criterion:
• Same as normal sinus rhythm except that the heart rate is slower than 60 beats/minute (thus increasing the risk of PVCs). Sinus bradycardia may be normal for your patient. In this case, no treatment is required. But if the condition is accompanied by hypotension or congestive heart failure, treatment is indicated.

Treatment
Patients with signs of poor cardiac output or heart failure may require one or more of the following measures:
• Give atropine, 0.4 mg I.V.
• Give I.V. isoproterenol (Isuprel), 0.2 to 1 mg in 250 to 500 ml dextrose 5% in water.
• For low output rates, the doctor will probably insert a temporary pacemaker. For irreversible symptoms of cardiac damage, he'll insert a permanent pacemaker.

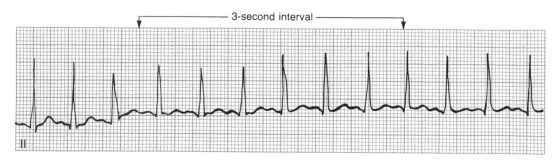

Sinus tachycardia

EKG criteria:
- Same as normal sinus rhythm except that the heart rate is between 100 and 160 beats/minute.
- P waves are sometimes difficult to see at higher heart rates, but they can usually be found on a 12-lead EKG.

Treatment
- Institute treatment of cause (for example: fever, anxiety, hypovolemia) if it can be determined.
- If heart disease had been diagnosed, watch for signs of congestive heart failure. To treat (or prevent) congestive heart failure, give digitalis and diuretics.

children and is associated with respiration — the variation of the sinus rate is related to normal inspiration and expiration. That is, it speeds up with inspiration and slows with expiration.

• *Sinus arrest.* Occasionally, the SA node will fail momentarily and will not initiate an impulse. This might be due to increased vagal stimulation (overeating, coffee, cigarettes), pharyngeal irritation (such as that caused by intubation), carotid sinus massage, or forced expiratory straining against a closed glottis (Valsalva's maneuver). This lack of impulse is called sinus arrest, although it is literally an atrial standstill. The atria are not stimulated to contract, so there is no atrial activity.

Sinus arrest may occur in patients who have received excess quantities of digitalis or quinidine. It is not usually of great importance to the patient unless he shows symptoms of fainting, dizziness, or syncope from the reduced cardiac output.

You can recognize sinus arrest on the EKG by the long pauses in which beats are dropped. That is, after a normal P wave and QRS complex, there will be no P wave but rather a pause (see middle EKG strip on opposite page). This may be followed by a normal P-QRS-T complex. Then the SA node again stimulates the atria.

When this dysrhythmia occurs, you should try to determine the cause. In most cases, you should watch the patient carefully for the side effects of poor cardiac output. If the patient has organic heart disease from myocardial irritation due to infection or infarction, an atrial pacemaker may be required. This may be either a permanent or temporary pacemaker, depending on the patient's prognosis and age.

• *Wandering pacemaker.* An often confusing dysrhythmia is the wandering pacemaker, in which the site of the impulse

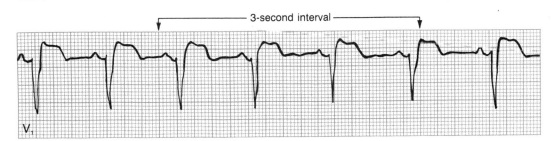

Sinus arrhythmia

EKG criteria:
- Same as normal sinus rhythm except PP intervals vary slightly.
- PR intervals vary slightly but within normal limits.

- Periods of slow and fast heart rates may alternate, especially in children, depending on crying or respirations.

Treatment
- None. But watch patients with variable PP intervals for premature atrial contractions and other atrial dysrhythmias.

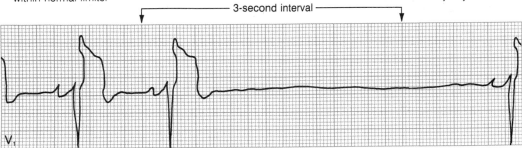

Sinus arrest (atrial standstill)

EKG criteria:
- Same as normal sinus rhythm except that an occasional long pause follows a regular beat (due to SA node failure to initiate impulse).
- PP interval is normal except that no P wave is seen during pause in cardiac rhythm.
- The pause is not a multiple of the normal PP interval.

Treatment
- Some patients require no treatment, depending on cause and effect of sinus arrest.
- If sinus arrest is due to car-diac damage near the SA node, the doctor will probably insert a temporary pacemaker.
- If SA node is unable to restore normal pacing, a permanent pacemaker may be needed.

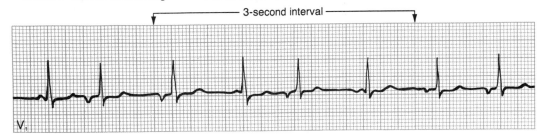

Wandering pacemaker

EKG criteria:
- P wave changes shape (configuration) and direction because of changing sites of pacing stimulus.

- PR interval varies from short to normal.
- Variations in rhythm occur because of changes in pacing stimulus.

Treatment
- If acute carditis is present, treat underlying infection.
- If due to digitalis excess, hold dosage for short period.

shifts. Sometimes beats originate in the SA node; other times they originate in an irritable atrial focus or even in the AV node.

Because the pacemaker site shifts, the P waves vary in configuration and direction and the PR intervals vary in length (see bottom EKG strip on previous page). Ventricular rhythm also varies slightly.

Wandering pacemaker may be caused by inflamed or irritated atrial tissue due to rheumatic carditis or other organic heart disease or by excesses of digitalis. Despite its unusual configuration, it is rarely serious.

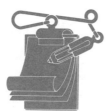

Remember these important points about SA node dysrhythmias:
1. Consider minute variations in the PP interval indicative of a sinus arrhythmia.
2. Be aware that a sinus rhythm is characterized by P waves of normal contour and a normal PR interval preceding each QRS complex.
3. Suspect sinus arrest when the EKG tracing shows long pauses in which beats are dropped and the pause is not a multiple of the normal PP interval.
4. When sinus arrest occurs, look for such possible causes as vagal stimulation, pharyngeal irritation, carotid sinus massage, or deep inspiration.
5. Observe the EKG tracing for P waves varying in configuration and direction, and PR intervals varying in length. If present, suspect a wandering pacemaker.

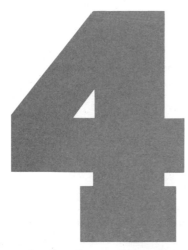

Atrial dysrhythmias:
Discretion in evaluation

As we noted in the last chapter, you would be mistaken to believe that the EKG can supply all the answers about a patient's condition, or even most of them. True, it provides data — valuable data. But only when interpreted in light of data from clinical observation, laboratory test results, and the patient's history can the EKG serve as a meaningful guide to treatment. This fact was occasionally apparent in our discussion of dysrhythmias of the SA node, such as sinus bradycardia. But it will become increasingly apparent in this chapter as we discuss atrial dysrhythmias.

A case in point is Dorothy's experience. Her complaint — that her heart was skipping beats — will sound familiar to any of you who have worked the E.D. or CCU. Dorothy was a 44-year-old nurse on our cardiac care staff. Her husband brought her to our E.D. at 2 o'clock one Sunday morning. Both she and her husband were thoroughly frightened, certain that she was having a heart attack.

The E.D. nurse took a brief history while preparing Dorothy for an EKG. Dorothy said she had never had any heart trouble nor could she recall any previous symptoms of cardiac problems before that night. She had been out for a late dinner, had

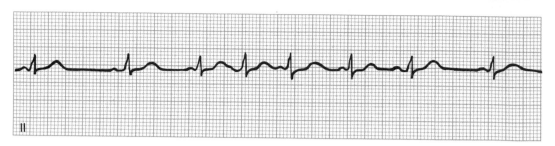

Dorothy's EKG*

drunk several cocktails and 3 or 4 cups of coffee, and had eaten much more heavily than normal. She had gone to bed about midnight, exhausted but relaxed. At 1:20 a.m. she awoke suddenly, acutely aware that her heartbeat was irregular. "I never noticed an irregular heartbeat before," she said. "I was afraid my heart would stop beating at any moment."

The E.D. nurse first ran a lead II rhythm strip, then checked it while the rest of the 12-lead EKG was being taken. A portion of lead II is shown above.

Based on the procedure you learned in Chapter 2, analyze the strip. As you work through the procedure, write your findings and then compare them with the criteria for premature atrial contractions (PACs) listed on the opposite page.

You should have found that, on Dorothy's rhythm strip, a P wave precedes each QRS complex, although one P wave is almost hidden in the preceding T wave. The P waves differ slightly in configuration. The RR interval becomes shorter in a few beats, but the QRS complex doesn't change configuration. The two beats following those with the shorter RR intervals (the PACs) don't occur at the expected time because the SA node — the heart's primary pacemaker — didn't reset itself or reestablish its timing. Therefore, these could also be considered PACs. Dorothy's diagnosis: normal sinus rhythm with many premature atrial contractions.

How should Dorothy be treated? The clue comes from her history. The premature beats were almost certainly caused by gastric overload plus alcohol and caffeine intake, all of which caused vagal stimulation. (Stimulating the vagus nerve slows the heart rate, leading to the PACs.) So, Dorothy was observed for a few hours and then sent home.

*Throughout the rest of this book, each small square on the EKG waveforms equals 0.04 second. Therefore, 15 of the larger blocks equals a 3-second interval.

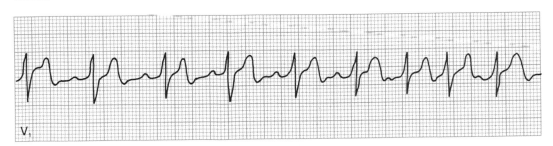

V₁

But suppose a patient on your nursing unit complained of skipping heartbeats. More than likely his EKG would look similar, but his treatment might differ because the PACs would have been caused by something different. For example, if your patient's receiving digitalis and he's experiencing atrial bigeminy (a normal sinus beat that alternates with a PAC), frequent PACs or clusters, he may have a low serum potassium level and digitalis toxicity. Or, he may also need more digitalis to make his serum level therapeutic.

But the patient with rheumatic carditis can also develop PACs. This is because the rheumatic disease process irritates the atrial myocardium.

Whatever the cause of the PACs, the patient should be monitored for signs of other dysrhythmias, such as atrial tachycardias, which often follow PACs. Unless they produce other dysrhythmias, PACs themselves are usually benign. Often they disappear without any treatment.

Obviously, the treatment of PACs differs markedly, according to the clinical circumstances. The same is true of many other dysrhythmias. As you read the following discussion of atrial dysrhythmias, remember that the availability of a cardiac monitor by no means relieves you of the responsibility of making careful nursing observations. The EKG tracing only provides additional data to be interpreted in light of your patient's history and clinical appearance.

Three atrial tachycardias

Three dysrhythmias are classified as atrial tachycardias. Each has a different mechanism, but all originate from atrial ectopic foci and have rates over 160 beats/minute.

• *Paroxysmal atrial tachycardia* (PAT) frequently occurs in healthy persons. In such cases it is benign. But when it occurs in a cardiac patient or in a patient who is critically ill, it can

Premature atrial contraction (PAC)
EKG criteria:
• Premature P wave may be lost in T wave.
• P wave may have abnormal configuration (flat, slurred, notched, inverted, diphasic, or wide).
• RR interval of premature beat is shorter than normal.
• PR interval may be longer or (occasionally) shorter than normal, depending on location of P wave.
• Pause following PAC is not usually compensatory (that is, the beat following premature beat doesn't occur at normal time because SA node timing was disturbed).
• QRS complex is normal, unless ventricular conduction is delayed or aberrant (follows a different or delayed pathway to ventricles).
Treatment
• Often no treatment is needed.
• If serum potassium is low, give P.O. or I.V. infusion of potassium.
• Give digitalis, as ordered, unless digitalis toxicity is the suspected cause of PACs.
• Give quinidine 200 mg, P.O., usually q.i.d., for patients with organic heart disease.
• Give propranolol if PACs occur in short runs of atrial tachycardia.

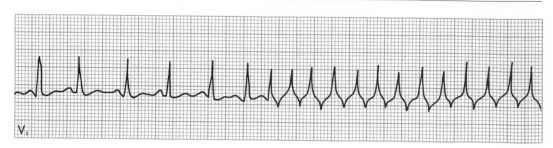

Paroxysmal atrial tachycardia (PAT)

EKG criteria:
- Ventricular beats/minute rhythm is perfectly regular with atrial rate of 160 to 250.
- QRS complex is usually narrow.
- P waves may have an abnormal contour or be difficult to see in any of the 12 leads.
- Onset is sudden, often initiated by PAC.

Treatment
- Have patient try Valsalva's maneuver.
- Apply carotid sinus pressure (only doctors do this).
- Give digitalis and verapamil. In some cases, propranolol (Inderal) is also effective.

be a forerunner of a more serious ventricular dysrhythmia.

PAT is a very rapid, regular heartbeat that begins suddenly and usually has been preceded by frequent PACs, one of which precipitates the tachycardia (shown above). In some cases, the tachycardia is brief; in others it lasts for hours. Often PAT begins while the patient is asleep, and the rapid beating awakens him.

A doctor may try one of two procedures to slow the rate. Either he'll ask the patient to breathe out forcefully and bear down (Valsalva's maneuver) or he'll use carotid sinus pressure. Either method stimulates the vagus nerve and slows impulse production at the SA and AV nodes, causing atrial standstill and giving the SA node a chance to reestablish itself as the main pacemaker. Then normal sinus rhythm is restored.

When the atrial rate is exactly twice the ventricular rate, the patient is said to have PAT with 2:1 block. This is a common sign of toxicity in digitalized patients.

Rapid rates can exhaust the patient, even those without organic disease. Therefore, you should watch the patient for signs of congestive heart failure. Be prepared to give an antiarrhythmic drug and diuretics, as ordered, and observe how they affect the patient and the dysrhythmia.

- *Atrial flutter* is an interesting dysrhythmia often misdiagnosed at PAT. As in PACs and PATs, the impulse comes from an atrial ectopic focus. Some cardiologists believe that the impulse derives from multiple ectopic foci (called *circus movement*), while others believe it derives from a single ectopic focus.

Atrial flutter rarely occurs in the absence of organic heart disease. Unless strictly controlled by the SA node, the atria move quickly and average 300 beats/minute. Actual atrial rates range from 250 to 350 beats/minute in patients with atrial flutter.

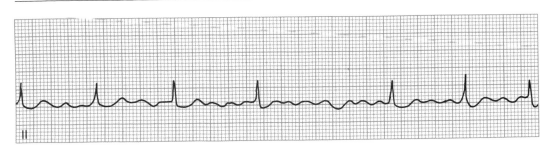

II

Because in this dysrhythmia atrial activity is so rapid, many of these impulses fail to pass through the AV node to the ventricles. Therefore, the atrial and ventricular rates differ greatly (for example: 300 atrial, 75 ventricular — a ratio of 4:1). The failure of ventricles to keep pace is fortunate, since rapid ventricular rates pose a threat to the patient. A lower ratio between atrial and ventricular rates (2:1 instead of 4:1) would more seriously threaten the patient because the ventricular rate would then be dangerously rapid.

In most cases of atrial flutter, the ventricular rhythm is very regular, but occasionally it is so irregular that you cannot establish a ratio between the atrial and ventricular rates (see above). An irregular ventricular rhythm often means the patient is getting ready to convert to atrial fibrillation, a favorable sign since in atrial fibrillation the ventricular rate is easier to control.

Most patients with atrial flutter respond to increased dosages of digitalis supplemented by propranolol hydrochloride (Inderal). This combination slows the impulses at the AV node, with the propranolol acting on the upper and lower nodal regions and digitalis affecting the midnodal region. As the ventricular rate slows, the atrial flutter may convert to atrial fibrillation, which can be treated, in turn, with quinidine and maintenance dosages of digitalis. In some cases, the flutter reverts directly to normal sinus rhythm. Atrial flutter can also be treated by cardioversion or atrial pacing with a temporary pacemaker.

At times, you may not be able to distinguish on the rhythm strip between atrial flutter and the dysrhythmia discussed on the next page — atrial fibrillation. These cases, representing either an impure flutter or a coarse fibrillation, are often referred to as "flutter-fib," or "fibro-flutter." Neither of these words are standard medical terminology, but they do ade-

Atrial flutter
EKG criteria:
- P waves are sawtoothed and referred to as flutter waves (F waves).
- QRS complex is usually narrow.
- Atrial rate is between 250 and 350 beats/minute; (usually 300/minute; determine rate by counting number of small squares between points of one sawtooth wave, then dividing into 1,500).
- Varying degrees of AV block (conduction) produce ventricular rates that are ½ to ¼ the atrial rate, giving ratios of 2:1, 3:1, and so forth.
- Ventricular rhythm, although usually regular, can be irregular because conduction ratio varies with each cycle.
- All flutter waves are uniform in width and proceed through QRS complex without interfering with either rhythm.

Treatment
Administer, as ordered, any of the following, either alone or in combination:
- Digitalis (unless flutter is due to digitalis toxicity)
- Propranolol
- Quinidine (after patient is digitalized)

The doctor may choose either of the following, if necessary:
- Elective cardioversion (if heart rate's greater than 300 beats/minute)
- Temporary atrial pacemaker

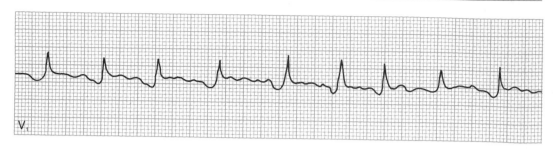

Atrial fibrillation

EKG criteria:
- Ventricular rhythm is completely irregular, with no pattern to irregularity.
- Atrial fibrillatory (f) waves may be superimposed on T waves.
- Atrial rate (determined as in atrial flutter) is between 350 and 500 beats/minute (could go as high as 700 beats/minute).
- No PR interval is visible.
- QRS complex is usually narrow unless conduction is delayed in ventricles.

Treatment
Administer, as ordered, any of the following, either alone or in combination:
- Digitalis, quinidine, or propranolol to slow ventricular rate and to convert to normal sinus rhythm
- Diuretics for congestive heart failure

The doctor may choose either of the following, if necessary:
- Elective cardioversion
- Temporary pacemaker for low ventricular rates due to AV block

quately describe the condition.

• *Atrial fibrillation* is easily recognized because of its grossly irregular ventricular rhythm. As with the other atrial dysrhythmias, the impulse originates in one or more irritable atrial ectopic areas. These ectopic foci discharge the irregular impulses at atrial rates as high as 500 or more beats/minute. Such a rapid rate creates a chaotic baseline, of varying shapes and sizes. Unlike atrial flutter, in which the flutter waves are uniform, the fibrillatory (or f) waves cause the atrial rate to constantly change through the tracing.

With such excitable, irregular atrial activity, the ventricles respond only to those impulses that pass through the AV node. This is a sporadic occurrence; so, in contrast to atrial flutter, the RR interval of atrial fibrillation is very irregular, with no pattern to the irregularity. In those cases when the ventricular rate is too rapid, propranolol or verapamil is added to the digitalis regimen to slow conduction through the AV node, thus slowing the ventricular response.

Some patients are admitted with the diagnosis of atrial fibrillation of unknown etiology. In many instances, despite the usual cardiac workup — 12-lead EKG, chest X-ray, cardiac enzyme and electrolyte studies, and continuous cardiac monitoring for several days — the etiology remains unknown. Such patients are usually discharged having had no dramatic treatment.

In fact, a large CCU will commonly have several patients in atrial fibrillation, each being treated differently. A striking example of this occurred in one hospital a while ago.

Same dysrhythmia, different treatments

One afternoon, George R. and Helen E., both in their early 40s, were admitted to the CCU. Both had a preliminary diagnosis of atrial fibrillation with *uncontrolled* ventricular rates.

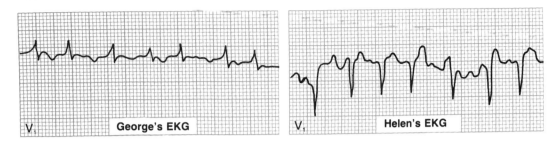

George's EKG   Helen's EKG

(Atrial fibrillation is *controlled* when the ventricular rate is below 100.) His was about 150 (see above left) and hers about 140 (see above right). The admitting nurse noted moist rales in both patients' chests, but George was dyspneic; his breath sounds were coarse.

After unsuccessful treatment with medications, George was prepared for elective cardioversion. His atrial rate was 500 beats/minute; his ventricular rate, 150. He was given nasal oxygen at 5 liters/minute for the dyspnea and furosemide (Lasix), 20 mg I.V., for the rales, which were becoming more pronounced. His response to the diuretic was fair.

Meanwhile, Helen was given digoxin, 0.25 mg stat I.V., and Lasix 10 mg I.V., to slow her heart rate and prevent congestive heart failure. An additional 0.25 mg dose of digoxin was given I.V. 2 hours later because her ventricular rate remained above 100 beats/minute. Oxygen, p.r.n., for dyspnea was also ordered.

Helen's urine output increased in response to the diuretic. After the first dose of digoxin, her ventricular rate slowed to 110; after the second dose, to 90. Her atrial fibrillation was controlled.

Why were these two patients, with the same dysrhythmia, treated so differently? Primarily, because the medical histories were vastly different.

George had a history of two previous myocardial infarctions, the last one complicated by severe congestive heart failure and episodes of PVCs. Because his myocardium was severely damaged, his increasingly irregular heart rate threatened to bring on congestive heart failure and a more lethal dysrhythmia.

After two shocks of 50 W/second each, the cardioversion restored his heart to a normal sinus rhythm of 86 beats/minute. He was then given digoxin, 0.25 mg orally b.i.d., and his

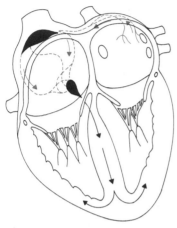

Pathway for atrial dysrhythmias
Impulses for atrial dysrhythmias originate outside the SA node, in either single or multiple ectopic foci.

daily Lasix dose was increased to 20 mg orally b.i.d. He was observed for 1 week and then discharged, doing well.

Helen had been hospitalized several times for evaluation and treatment of mitral stenosis. Her ventricular myocardium was undamaged, so we knew we had time to observe her and could treat her more conservatively. Besides, in patients with mitral stenosis and atrial fibrillation, cardioversion increases the risk of an embolus from left atrial clots (commonly found in patients with mitral stenosis).

Hospitalized for 3 weeks, she underwent successful open-heart surgery for her mitral stenosis. When discharged she still had atrial fibrillation with a ventricular rate of 76 — not a serious problem for her. Cardioversion was not attempted post-operatively because a patient with long-standing fibrillation with mitral stenosis isn't likely to return to sinus rhythm.

Upon discharge, Helen was doing well on medication — digoxin, 0.25 mg, and hydrochlorothiazide, 50 mg daily.

The most important thing to remember is that the seriousness of a dysrhythmia can be judged only in the context of its meaning to the patient. This is where you, the nurse, come in. Who can better judge the patient's changes in condition? You know how the patient looks, and if there were any changes in his appearance. You have access to his history, his care plans, his chart, and all the information pertaining to his condition. You must consider all of this information before you can determine what action, if any, is required when changes occur in the patient's rhythm strip or in his condition.

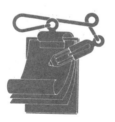

Remember these important points about atrial dysrhythmias:
1. Consider a patient with a history of heart disease, especially rheumatic carditis, at high risk of developing premature atrial contractions (PACs).
2. Monitor the patient with PACs for other signs of dysrhythmias, such as atrial tachycardias.
3. Keep in mind that atrial tachycardias originate from the atrial ectopic foci and have rates over 160 beats/minute.
4. Watch the patient with paroxysmal atrial tachycardia (PATs) for signs of congestive heart failure. Be ready to give antiarrhythmics and diuretics, as ordered.
5. Assess the dysrhythmia's severity by the patient's appearance, health history, care plan, and chart.

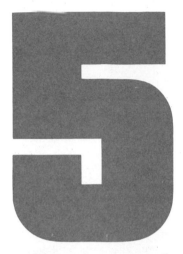

Junctional dysrhythmias:
A cause for disquiet

Watching an EKG tracing emerge from the machine, you sometimes feel your anxiety rising. Being a professional, you don't let it show. But you're also human; you cannot avoid reacting emotionally to evidence on that rhythm strip suggesting that your patient is a lot sicker than imagined.

In the next three chapters, we'll be discussing dysrhythmias capable of raising a nurse's anxiety level: junctional dysrhythmias, AV blocks, ventricular dysrhythmias, and bundle branch blocks. All of these differ from the sinus arrhythmias and atrial dysrhythmias discussed earlier by one outstanding feature: sinus arrhythmias and atrial dysrhythmias (except for atrial flutter) may appear in healthy people; junctional dysrhythmias, AV blocks, ventricular dysrhythmias, and bundle branch blocks rarely occur in healthy people — and they're almost always serious.

Even though junctional dysrhythmias are generally regarded as the least dangerous of this group, they are serious and call for prompt treatment.

What causes junctional dysrhythmias?
Normally, the SA node is the heart's pacemaker. However,

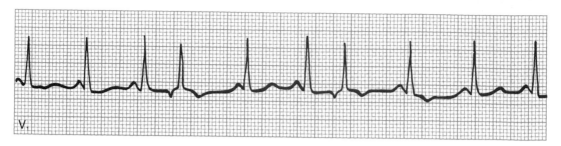

Premature nodal contraction
EKG criteria:
- RR interval of premature beat is shorter than the patient's normal interval.
- PR interval is short (less than 0.12 second).
- P wave inverts in leads II, III, and aVF, and is upright in aVR and aVL.
- P wave may be before QRS complex, lost in QRS complex, or follow QRS complex and be inverted.

Treatment
- Give potassium supplement if indicated.
- Give digitalis, quinidine, or procainamide if junctional premature beats occur frequently (more than 6/minute).
- If digitalis toxicity is suspected, digitalis should be discontinued.

the AV node takes over this role in certain cases of organic heart disease, atrial ischemia, myocardial infarction, or over-digitalization.

When the AV node assumes the pacemaker role, *junctional dysrhythmias* result. The impulse originating in the AV node travels first to the ventricles, then rebounds to stimulate the atria. Called *retrograde conduction*, this mechanism may diminish cardiac output, especially when the ventricular rate is very slow or very rapid.

Consequently, junctional dysrhythmias are serious. Most commonly, they occur in patients who have organic heart disease; in some cases, they lead to congestive heart failure.

- *Premature beats.* If the AV node takes over as the dominant pacemaker for only one beat, it is called a *junctional premature beat* or a *premature nodal contraction (PNC).* Such a condition can be caused by an excess of digitalis or an excess of quinidine.

You can differentiate between a premature atrial contraction (PAC) and a junctional premature beat by the location of the P wave. In a PAC, the RR interval is shorter than normal and the P wave may appear closer to or as part of the T wave, making the PR interval longer. In a PNC (shown above), the RR interval also is shorter than normal. But the P wave may be closer to, be lost in, or follow the QRS complex, making the PR interval short (less than 0.12 second).

Sometimes, though, the P wave may be so indistinct that you can't tell whether it's a PAC or a PNC. What do you do then? That's when you have to make a judgment based on the patient's history and diagnosis. Does he have rheumatic carditis, for example — a common cause of PACs? Or does he have organic heart disease — common in patients with PNCs? Is his serum potassium level low, as it often is with PACs? Answers to all of these questions should help give you some

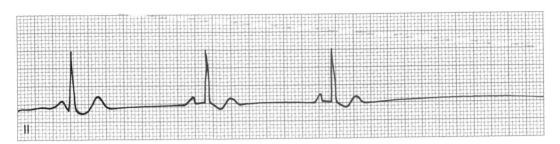

clues to the patient's problem.

Still, there are times when the answers don't help — no one can determine whether a patient has PACs or PNCs. All that can be said for certain is that the impulse originates above the bifurcation of the bundle of His. Since the exact origin of these beats is unknown, they are called *supraventricular premature beats*.

Whatever the origin of the premature beat, you must stay alert for other developing dysrhythmias. If any arise, immediately report them to the doctor. If the patient's serum potassium level is low, the doctor may order an I.V. potassium infusion; often, that's enough to eliminate the premature beats. If the patient has ventricular damage (such as myocardial infarction), the doctor may order quinidine or procainamide by mouth to quell or prevent ventricular irritability.

• *Nodal rhythms.* If the AV node takes over as the dominant pacemaker for a succession of beats, the patient is in *nodal rhythm* or *nodal tachycardia*. Usually, the AV node can initiate impulses of from 40 to 60 beats/minute, the so-called *junctional* (or *nodal*) *rhythm* (shown above). A junctional rhythm of more than 60 beats/minute is called *junctional tachycardia* (see EKG strip on next page). Junctional tachycardia may be either slow (under 100 beats/minute) or rapid (over 100 beats/minute). A junctional tachycardia of sudden onset, called *paroxysmal junctional tachycardia*, (150 to 220 beats/minute), usually indicates digitalis toxicity.

The terms nodal, junctional, and AV junctional dysrhythmia are used interchangeably; all refer to a dysrhythmia originating in the AV node. To further complicate terminology, many electrocardiographers and textbooks refer to a specific section of the AV node in diagnosing a dysrhythmia. Anatomically, the AV node is divided into upper, middle, and lower nodal regions. The upper nodal region borders on the atria; the lower,

Junctional (nodal) rhythm
EKG criteria:
• P wave precedes QRS complex, but PR interval is shorter than 0.11 second. (P wave could be inverted in leads II and III.)
• Or P wave, lost in QRS complex, is not visible.
• Or P wave follows QRS complex and is inverted (retrograde conduction).
• QRS duration is normal unless conduction is aberrant.
• Ventricular rate is between 40 and 60 beats/minute.
Treatment
• If digitalis is suspected as cause, discontinue it.
• Atropine may be indicated.
• Give diuretic to prevent or control congestive heart failure.
• Temporary pacemaker may need to be inserted if cardiac output is poor.

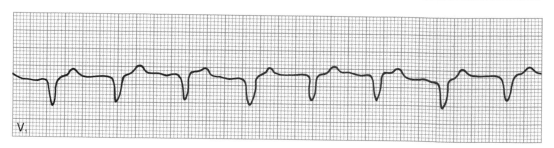

Junctional (nodal) tachycardia

EKG criteria:

- Same P wave location and QRS complex as in junctional rhythm.
- Ventricular rate is 60 to 100 beats/minute (slow) or 100 to 220 beats/minute (rapid). (Rapid junctional tachycardia of sudden onset is paroxysmal junctional tachycardia.)

Treatment

- If digitalis toxicity is the cause (likely in paroxysmal junctional tachycardia), withhold dosage and give diuretic to prevent congestive heart failure.
- The doctor may use carotid massage to terminate rapid nodal tachycardia.
- Give propranolol.
- Give phenytoin.
- Give potassium chloride I.V. with I.V. fluids, if ordered.

on the bundle of His. (This entire region is also referred to as the junctional region.)

An upper nodal dysrhythmia can be identified by a short PR interval, with a P wave that may be inverted preceding the QRS complex. In a midnodal dysrhythmia, the P wave may be "riding" or entirely lost in the QRS complex. A low nodal dysrhythmia is identified by an inverted P wave following the QRS complex. At times, you may not be able to determine whether the dysrhythmia, like a single premature junctional contraction, is derived from an impulse originating in the low atrial region or the upper nodal region. Although in such cases the point of origin is not precisely known, it is known to be located above the ventricles; hence the resulting disturbance or dysrhythmia is classified simply as a *supraventricular dysrhythmia.*

A case in point

Whatever the specific origin of impulse, a junctional dysrhythmia poses real danger to the patient, as the following example illustrates.

Rosemary P., a 35-year-old mother of three, came to our ICU immediately after her third operation for mitral valve disease. This time the surgeon implanted a St. Jude mitral valve prosthesis, and we hoped it would see her through many good years. Since most of us had been on the unit when Rosemary had had her previous operations, we considered her almost part of the family. We wanted to make this postop period as easy as possible for her.

Although concerned about the usual postop heart surgery complications, which included shock, hemorrhage, and stroke from emboli, we were even more concerned about the possibility of a serious dysrhythmia. We'd have been surprised if Rosemary had maintained the normal sinus rhythm she had

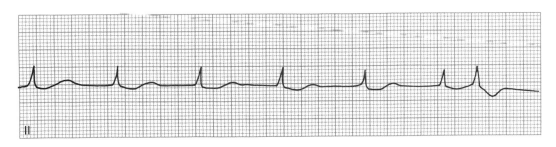

Rosemary's EKG

upon return from the O.R. Like most mitral patients, she'd had atrial fibrillation for years, so we expected her to revert to it soon.

Midmorning of Rosemary's first postop day, her rhythm on the monitor changed abruptly to a slow junctional tachycardia, with premature ventricular contractions (PVCs) close to the T wave. We did a stat EKG to confirm the junctional pacing, then looked for better P waves, especially in leads II and V_1.

A portion of Rosemary's rhythm strip is shown above. Can you analyze it? Compare your analysis with the criteria for junctional rhythm and junctional tachycardia (see pages 51 and 52).

Notice the absense of P waves. Clearly, the impulse could not be coming from the SA node. The PVC's proximity to the T wave of the preceding beat is another danger sign, which we'll discuss in Chapter 7.

What caused Rosemary's dysrhythmia? We suspected digitalis. Since surgery, she had been given a total of only 1 mg of digoxin — not an excessive dosage for a postop patient with mitral valve disease. However, if hypokalemia were present, digitalis toxicity could still have been responsible. Another likely cause was the heart's inflammation and edema resulting from the recent surgery.

Besides keeping a close watch on her EKG, we watched Rosemary for signs of congestive heart failure, listening to her lungs for moist rales and carefully checking her fluid intake and output as well as vital signs.

As a precaution, we withheld further digitalis. As ordered, we added 40 mEq of potassium chloride to the day's I.V. fluids (a total of 1,000 ml) because her serum potassium level was 3.9. Although this is not dangerously low, hypokalemia could have contributed to the dysrhythmia.

Because of Rosemary's cardiac history and the PVCs, the

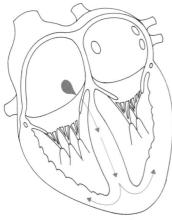

Pathway for junctional dysrhythmias
When the AV node assumes the pacemaker role, junctional dysrhythmias result.

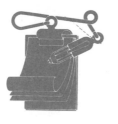

doctor ordered quinidine, 200 mg every 6 hours by mouth. Quinidine quiets both the atrial and ventricular myocardial irritability, and the PVCs soon disappeared. The junctional rate held steady at 70 — a slow junctional tachycardia.

Midafternoon of the second postop day, Rosemary converted to atrial fibrillation with a ventricular rate of 84. The PVCs had not recurred, so we continued the quinidine until after discharge. (Quinidine is commonly used prophylactically on patients with conditions similar to Rosemary's.) As ordered, we restarted digoxin, 0.25 mg, on the third postop day, and Rosemary had no further dysrhythmias during the remainder of her hospitalization.

In one respect, Rosemary was fortunate. Her ventricular rate with the junctional dysrhythmia never exceeded 70. In a dysrhythmia caused by digitalis toxicity, the ventricular rate could have increased to as high as 220 beats/minute. Such rapid rates greatly decrease cardiac output, which could be fatal to a patient in Rosemary's condition.

Although not needed in Rosemary's case, in many cases propranolol is used to reverse paroxysmal junctional tachycardia.

Remember these important points about junctional dysrhythmias:
1. Watch for junctional dysrhythmias in patients with organic heart disease, atrial ischemia, myocardial infarction, or overdigitalization.
2. Differentiate between an atrial beat and a junctional premature beat by determining P wave presence, location, and shape.
3. Identify an upper nodal dysrhythmia by its short PR interval and the P wave preceding the QRS complex, which may be inverted.
4. When your patient's ventricular rate becomes abnormally rapid (60 to 100 beats/minute), suspect digitalis toxicity.
5. Be aware that low serum potassium levels may cause premature beats.

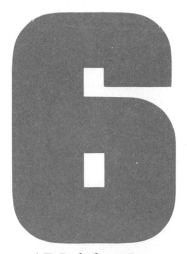

AV blocks:
The value of a suspicious mind

By now you should realize that EKG interpretation involves a lot more than a few technical skills. No doubt you've found it takes something closer to the artistry of a practiced sleuth: a sharp eye for detail and the persistence to explore all possible interpretations. In addition, it takes a suspicious mind — a developed instinct to suspect the worst possible explanation and then to try to disprove it. If your worst suspicion proves incorrect, you can still test for less serious conditions. But if your worst suspicion proves correct, you'll be on top of the situation and have plenty of time to correct it.

The value of a suspicious mind underlies all EKG interpretation, but it is especially important with AV blocks. As many tragic stories attest, too often nurses glance only at the monitor and so mistake these dangerous dysrhythmias for a sinus bradycardia or a sinus arrhythmia. They fail to check the rhythm strip. So, while they go on to examine the rhythm strip of another patient with a serious problem, the patient with the AV block may progress to ventricular asystole.

AV block
Any conduction disturbance in the heart is referred to as a

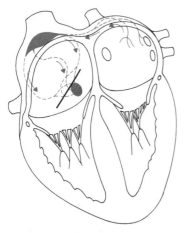

Pathway of AV blocks
Although the impulse originates
in the SA node, an abnormality in
the AV node blocks it.

block. The most common are AV blocks — conduction delays in the AV node — which are classified as first-degree AV block, second-degree AV block (Mobitz Type I, or Wencke-bach, and Mobitz Type II), and third-degree AV block (complete heart block).

We can also classify blocks according to cause. AV blocks may be caused by excessive doses of such drugs as digitalis or quinidine; by myocardial infarction or degeneration of conduction tissue due to age; by a suture that is inadvertently placed through the AV node during open heart surgery, resulting in impaired atrioventricular conduction; and, following open heart surgery, by manipulation or by edema in the nodal region resulting in damage (usually temporary) to nodal tissue.

Sometimes the AV node is refractory to an impulse — it doesn't or can't permit the impulse to pass directly through it. In this case, repolarization must occur before an impulse is permitted to travel to the ventricles. If the block is due to injury, further evaluation of the degree of blockage is required and appropriate therapy instituted.

As with the dysrhythmias discussed earlier, you can gain insight into the location and type of block from the EKG; but to decide on appropriate treatment, you must know the cause of the block and the patient's response to it. You might have two patients on your unit with second-degree AV block. One might require immediate treatment, the other only close observation. What treatment, if any, is required would depend primarily on the deterioration in cardiac output resulting from the dysrhythmia.

An asymptomatic patient is apt to require only observation; very likely no symptoms will develop and no treatment may be needed. On the other hand, the onset of syncope or convulsions would point to severe block with a very slow ventricular rate, requiring immediate treatment. The treatment might consist of temporary pacing with a demand pacemaker to improve cardiac function. The temporary pacing will give you time to observe how much pacing your patient requires, to decide when and if he will require permanent pacing, and to teach him how to live with a permanent pacemaker if it's needed.

A less aggressive treatment for patients with low output and AV blocks is atropine therapy, which increases atrial contractility by speeding the rate of the sinus node. If the AV node

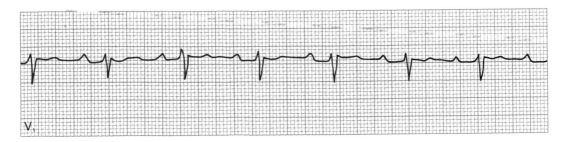

is not too badly damaged, the atropine improves the conduction of impulses to the ventricles. As a result, your patient's cardiac output is improved.

First-degree AV block

The most common conduction disturbance, first-degree AV block, can occur in apparently healthy persons as well as in those with diseased hearts. First-degree block is usually clinically insignificant; certainly it is considered less dangerous than the other types of blocks.

Chronic degeneration of the conduction system causes first-degree block in many elderly patients without evidence of heart disease. Antiarrhythmic drugs, such as digitalis, are another cause of first-degree block. In children, acute rheumatic fever may be the cause; indeed, first-degree block may be the earliest sign of the disease.

In first-degree AV block, impulses are conducted normally from the SA node through the atria but are delayed when they reach the AV node. You can recognize the block on the EKG above: each P wave is followed by a QRS complex, but the PR interval is prolonged — 0.20 second or longer. Although generally constant, the PR intervals may vary slightly if the heart rate changes significantly. In some instances, the PR interval may be as long as 0.70 to 0.80 second. Then the P wave may be fused with the preceding T wave, resembling an AV nodal rhythm. When the PR interval is exceptionally long, you should also suspect hidden P waves, which may signify second-degree AV block. You'll need to carefully inspect the full 12-lead EKG to detect the P wave before you can make a decision.

By itself, first-degree AV block does not significantly affect cardiac output. But if a patient's myocardium is already severely damaged, the block may advance to a more serious

First-degree AV heart block
EKG criterion:
* PR interval is prolonged beyond 0.20 second.
Treatment
* In most cases, none.

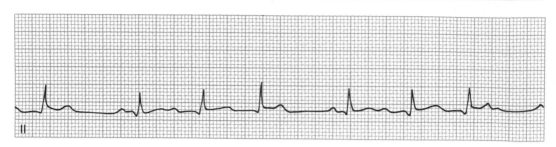

II

Second-degree AV heart block: Mobitz Type I (Wenckebach)

EKG criteria:
- PR interval becomes longer with each cycle until a P wave lacks a succeeding QRS complex. (Beat drops because of block.)
- RR interval gets progressively shorter (despite prolonged PR interval).
- RR interval containing blocked QRS complex is shorter than intervals of two normal sinus cycles.
- PR interval after the dropped beat is shorter than the one before.
- Blocked beats (dropped QRS complex) are usually cyclic in that a ratio can be established; for example, 3 P waves to 2 QRS complexes = 3:2 ratio (3 impulses, 2 conductions).

Treatment
- Temporary pacemaker may need to be inserted if patient experiences such symptoms as hypotension and/or syncope.

state because of the damage to or near the conduction system.

Second-degree AV block

There are two types of second-degree AV block: Mobitz Type I (or Wenckebach) and Mobitz Type II. Both types are characterized by occasional dropped ventricular beats. On the EKG, this will show up as a series of normal cycles, followed by a P wave without a QRS complex. Dropped beats mean that the impulse was conducted through the atria, but its passage through the AV node was blocked. Generally, in second-degree AV block the AV conduction ratio is 3:2 or 4:3, indicating that two out of three or three out of four impulses are conducted to the ventricles.

In most cases, the Mobitz Type I (Wenckebach) AV block occurs in patients who have an inferior wall myocardial infarction or digitalis toxicity. Often a transient dysrhythmia, it may also be caused by acute rheumatic fever, electrolyte imbalance, vagal stimulation, and occasionally by quinidine or procainamide therapy.

In the Mobitz Type I block (shown above), the PR interval is normal or even short when it begins, but gets longer and longer with each cycle until finally a QRS complex is dropped. Then the cycle begins again.

Here's what happens: The AV node's diseased conducting tissues become fatigued more easily than normal tissues. Conduction of each impulse causes greater fatigue, so each sinus impulse is conducted more and more slowly (prolonging the PR interval). Finally, the tissues become so fatigued that they are not able to conduct the sinus impulse at all; passage through the AV node is thus blocked. But this also gives the AV node a chance to rest, so it can conduct the next impulse in the normal time.

Less commonly, a Mobitz Type I block may have only one

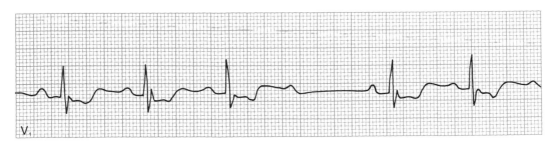

nonconducted P wave between long periods of normally conducted P waves. Then the progression of the prolonged PR interval may be so slight that it will be difficult to detect.

In Mobitz Type I block, the ventricular rhythm is slightly irregular because the RR intervals become progressively shorter despite the prolonged PR interval. The atrial rhythm, however, usually remains regular.

If the patient is asymptomatic, the prognosis is good for this Mobitz Type I second-degree block. In most cases, this block doesn't significantly affect cardiac output because the ventricular rate remains nearly normal.

Mobitz Type II AV block (shown above) is less common than Mobitz Type I but is also more serious, occurring in patients with acute myocardial infarction or severe coronary artery disease. Many times, it progresses to third-degree or complete block, requiring permanent pacing.

Type II resembles Type I in that both are characterized by dropped QRS complexes, but in Type II the PR and RR intervals do not vary. In other words, the dropped beat occurs completely without warning, in contrast to the prolonged PR interval that signals an impending dropped beat in Mobitz Type I block.

You can determine the seriousness of either type of second-degree block by the width of the QRS complex. If the QRS complex is narrow, the block is higher in the AV node and is less dangerous to the patient. If the QRS complex is wide, the block is farther down in the conduction system — usually below the bundle of His or near the bundle branches. The latter indicates more damaged cardiac tissue, often including the bundle branches; it is much more dangerous to the patient as it could produce Stokes-Adams syndrome. Hence, permanent pacing will probably be required.

Second-degree AV heart block: Mobitz Type II (4:3 block)
EKG criteria:
- PR interval is constant.
- QRS complex is periodically dropped after a P wave. (Beat is dropped because of block.)
- QRS complex is wide.

Treatment
- Temporary pacemaker and, eventually, permanent pacemaker may need to be inserted if patient experiences such symptoms as hypotension and/or syncope.

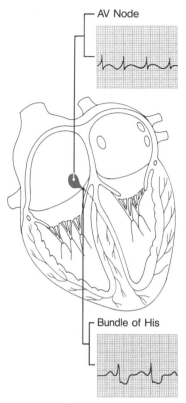

AV Node

Bundle of His

QRS: An important clue
To pinpoint a heart block's location, study the QRS complex.
If the block occurs high in the junctional region (AV node), the QRS complex will be narrow.
If the block occurs lower in the junctional region (bundle of His), the QRS complex will be wide. This conduction delay may progress to a higher grade of AV block and eventually lead to syncope or congestive heart failure.

Another type of second-degree AV block that must be considered separately is 2:1 AV block. In 2:1 AV block, every second sinus or atrial impulse is blocked, which means every other QRS complex is dropped. Therefore, each QRS complex is associated with two P waves. If 2:1 block occurs by itself, it's almost impossible to determine whether it is Mobitz Type I or II because you cannot determine the PR interval. Since you cannot determine if it is prolonged, you'll have to observe the rhythm and the patient for signs of improvement or deterioration. With that information, you should be able to classify the block.

Third-degree AV block

In third-degree AV block (complete heart block), the atria and ventricles act independently of each other, each producing its own impulses. This occurs because a complete block at the AV junction prevents all the impulses produced in the SA node from passing through to the ventricles. So, the ventricles must initiate their own impulse; the ventricular rate is then determined by the block's location and the origin of the subsidiary impulse.

If the block occurs high in the AV node, the subsidiary pacemaker will be below the blocked area but still high (above the bundle of His). The ventricular rate will be 45 to 60 beats/minute — slightly slower than normal sinus rhythm. In these instances the QRS complex will be narrow.

If the block occurs lower in the AV junction, the subsidiary pacemaker will be below the bundle of His, perhaps in the bundle branches, and the ventricular rate will be between 30 and 40 beats/minute. Here the QRS complex will be wide. These rates of less than 40 beats/minute are also called *idioventricular rhythms* since they arise in lower portions of the AV node or the ventricles. Rates this slow impair cardiac output and thus pose a danger to the patient.

In patients with third-degree block, the atrial rate is faster than the ventricular rate (see EKG strip on next page). The atrial impulse may originate in the SA node, producing normal sinus rhythm; or it may originate in an atrial ectopic focus, producing atrial tachycardia, atrial flutter, or atrial fibrillation.

In some cases complete block is due to digitalis toxicity. Such dysrhythmias are likely to be transient, and the ventricular rate is likely to be rapid enough to prevent syncope or

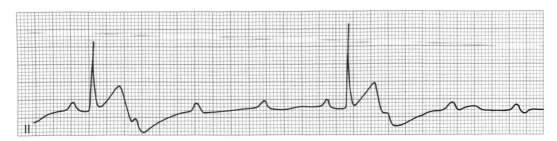

congestive heart failure. Beyond discontinuing digitalis and observing for signs of impaired cardiac output, many patients require no treatment; others require a temporary pacemaker.

In other cases, third-degree AV block may be congenital — or it may be caused by acute rheumatic fever, acute myocardial infarction, or diffuse fibrosis throughout the conduction system. It may also occur after open-heart surgery, especially in patients with septal defects.

If the block is congenital, it probably will not cause symptoms and no pacing is required despite the slow ventricular rates. The reason for this is not well understood. In contrast, an acquired complete block almost always produces symptoms, such as Stokes-Adams syncope, severe congestive heart failure, and ventricular irritability (PVCs or runs of ventricular tachycardia).

Complete block in a patient with acute myocardial infarction may be either transient or permanent, depending on the amount of myocardial damage and the subsidiary pacemaker site. For example, if a patient with acute inferior myocardial infarction develops complete block with a ventricular rate exceeding 50 beats/minute and has no signs of congestive heart failure, he may only require monitoring and, possibly, small doses of atropine. If the patient develops a ventricular rate below 40 beats/minute, hypotension, or congestive heart failure, a temporary pacemaker may be inserted. Normal AV conduction usually returns within 5 to 7 days. But slow heart rates predispose to PVCs (rule of bigeminy) and runs of ventricular tachycardia.

In contrast, a patient with anterior wall myocardial infarction who develops complete block usually has symptoms: either syncope or congestive heart failure. Because the myocardium is severely damaged, a permanent pacemaker probably must be inserted. Even so, damage to the anterior

Third-degree AV heart block (complete heart block)
EKG criteria:
- Atrial and ventricular rates differ. Atrial rate is faster than ventricular rate.
- P waves are not related to QRS complexes; they do not indicate ventricular contraction from a sinus beat because impulse is not conducted to ventricles (AV dissociation).
- PR interval varies.

Treatment
- Insertion of permanent pacemaker will probably be necessary.
- Stop digitalis.

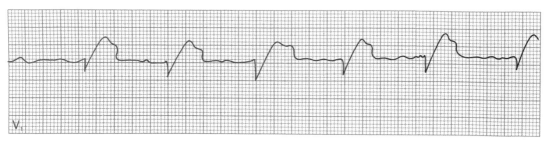

Jim's EKG at admission

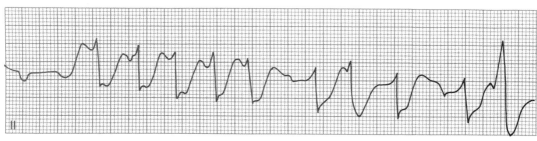

Jim's EKG at 9:00 p.m.

wall implies a poor prognosis, as illustrated by the following example.

AV block resulting from infarction

While at work, Jim C., a 42-year-old advertising executive, had a sudden, sharp, stabbing pain in his chest that radiated down his left arm. He was brought to our hospital by the police emergency rescue squad. Within minutes after his arrival, he was admitted to our coronary care unit.

Jim's history was typical. He had a high-pressure job and frequently suffered bouts of chest discomfort, fatigue, and indigestion. His family had a history of coronary disease, hypertension, and diabetes, and Jim himself was a heavy smoker, overweight, and hypertensive.

Suspecting a myocardial infarction, we gave him a complete medical workup, including laboratory and X-ray studies. Meanwhile, we treated him as an MI patient according to our CCU routine.

We ran a stat 12-lead EKG and initiated cardiac monitoring. We also started an I.V., and drew blood for measuring cardiac enzymes and arterial blood gases and for routine studies. We started nasal oxygen and gave him morphine, 5 mg I.V., as

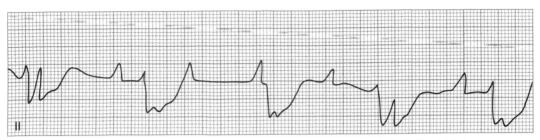

Jim's EKG at 9:03 p.m.

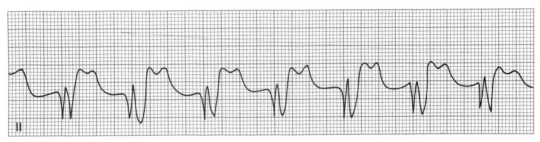

Jim's EKG after pacemaker insertion

needed, for the recurring pain. Looking at Jim's EKG strip at admission (see opposite page), can you analyze it?

Jim had a slow sinus rhythm at a rate of 60 beats/minute and his PR interval was slightly prolonged at 0.24 second, indicating first-degree AV block. The ST segment is elevated, indicating anterior wall ischemia. These EKG changes plus his pain and history led us to suspect that Jim would soon progress to an anterior wall infarction. We watched closely for additional dysrhythmias (particularly PVCs or a higher degree of block). We knew that the slow rate could cause congestive heart failure, but it had not yet caused any symptoms.

We monitored Jim's EKG, fluid balance, vital signs, breath sounds, and clinical picture. We looked for signs of congestive heart failure or deterioration in cardiac status. That evening about 7:00, Jim's QRS complex widened to 0.16 second, but his heart rate was 60 beats/minute. The PR interval increased to 0.32 second. Then everything seemed to happen at once.

At 9:00, Jim developed a short run of ventricular tachycardia (see opposite page) quickly followed by complete heart block with a ventricular rate of 44 (see top EKG strip above). Conduction to the ventricles had deteriorated and his condition was critical. He became diaphoretic and restless. His blood pressure fell to 90/60. His urine output decreased. Then he began to have frequent PVCs. After a lidocaine bolus of 50 mg, we started a lidocaine drip, as ordered. However, with AV block, lidocaine must be administered cautiously because it may further increase the degree of block, even though it suppresses the PVCs.

Jim was in cardiogenic shock. A temporary demand pacemaker set for 75 beats/minute was inserted. (Since pacemakers are common treatment for some dysrhythmias, you should be able to recognize the distinctive EKG features they produce — a widened QRS complex and a pacemaker spike before the QRS complex; see bottom EKG strip on previous page.) Jim's PVCs disappeared, his blood pressure rose to 110/70, and his general condition improved. Although the doctor may have ordered Isuprel, Aramine, dopamine, epinephrine, or Levophed to raise his blood pressure, the pacemaker was chosen because of the severity of shock and the presence of complete heart block. For the next several hours, Jim's condition remained stable.

The next morning, shortly after the change of shift, Jim developed intense chest pain and, in quick succession, PVCs, ventricular fibrillation, and cardiac arrest. Our efforts to resuscitate him failed.

An autopsy revealed that the blood supply to the anterior and some of the posterior myocardium was completely cut off, resulting in a massive, lethal infarction of the left ventricle. This also caused the dysrhythmias that preceded death. Nothing would have restored Jim's health — his disease was too advanced.

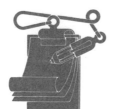

Remember these important points about AV blocks:
1. When a patient develops syncope or hypotension, suspect a severe block requiring immediate treatment.
2. Consider atropine therapy a less aggressive treatment for patients with low output and AV blocks. Atropine increases atrial contractility by speeding the rate of the sinus node.
3. In children, be aware that first-degree AV block may be an early sign of acute rheumatic fever.
4. Look for a Mobitz Type I AV block in a patient who has an inferior wall myocardial infarction or digitalis toxicity.
5. Know that a wide QRS complex indicates the more clinically serious Mobitz Type II AV block.

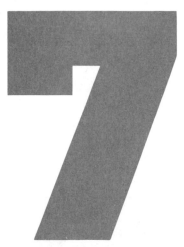

Ventricular dysrhythmias:
Possible exceptions

In the preceding chapters, we've stressed the importance of considering your patient's whole picture — his history, clinical observations, laboratory data, and so forth — before judging the seriousness of the dysrhythmia and determining what nursing interventions, if any, might be required. But with ventricular dysrhythmias, the EKG is the best means of recognizing the dysrhythmia and determining its seriousness.

Ventricular dysrhythmias are almost always serious. They may occur suddenly and are often rapidly fatal despite vigorous treatment. On the other hand, like the dysrhythmias discussed in earlier chapters, they are occasionally benign, as the following case illustrates.

Harold S., a 29-year-old pharmaceutical representative, went to his doctor for a routine physical examination. Much to his and the doctor's surprise, Harold's EKG showed ectopic ventricular activity, as indicated by premature ventricular contractions (PVCs). Consequently, the family doctor referred him to a cardiologist, who admitted him to the hospital and placed him on CCU telemetry for observation.

Despite the low incidence of myocardial infarction in men under 30, we considered this a possibility but quickly ruled it

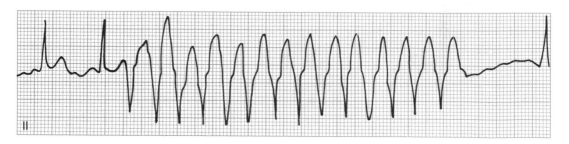

Harold's EKG at admission

out based on Harold's history, laboratory data, EKG, and physical examination.

Continuous cardiac monitoring showed that Harold did indeed have frequent episodes of ectopic ventricular activity — that is PVCs followed by short runs of ventricular tachycardia (see above). Each time we saw the tachycardia on the monitor, we'd run to Harold's room only to find him resting quietly or even asleep. When awake he felt no ill effects from the disturbance. Yet he was aware of it; he'd stop in the middle of a conversation to tell us, "It's happening again," then go on speaking as though everything were normal.

The doctor ordered various drugs — lidocaine, quinidine, and procainamide — but none of them had any effect on the dysrhythmias. After several days of observation, with still no success with drug therapy, Harold underwent cardiac catheterization for a suspected cardiomyopathy. But his coronary angiography and the rest of his catheterization data showed no cardiac damage. An exercise tolerance test showed that during exercise his PVCs disappeared as did the ventricular tachycardia. Repeated Holter monitoring and stress tests also confirmed the disappearance of the PVCs.

Eventually, Harold was discharged on propranolol, 10 mg t.i.d., which partially controlled the ventricular tachycardia. He appears to be living a full and normal life without any serious effects from his dysrhythmia.

Harold's case is not so unusual. Why didn't he have any ill effects from a dysrhythmia that in most patients would be considered ominous? As with the dysrhythmias discussed earlier, the answer lies in the effect on cardiac output. Harold had good peripheral perfusion despite his PVCs and tachycardia. Even as the PVCs appeared on his monitor, his pulse became only slightly weaker. Had we been unable to feel the pulse when we saw a PVC, we'd have known that the ven-

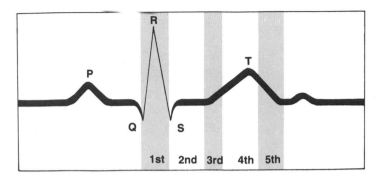

Depolarization-repolarization cycle
The ventricular depolarization-repolarization cycle consists of five periods:
1. Normal excitable period
2. Absolute refractory period
3. Relative refractory period
4. Vulnerable period
5. Supernormal period

tricular contractions were unable to maintain cardiac output.

Varieties of PVCs

PVCs *may* occur in seemingly healthy persons like Harold. They are more common, though, when the heart is diseased or injured. They occur rarely in a child or infant, commonly in a 50-year-old cardiac patient, usually in a person over 70.

PVCs originate in an ectopic focus of the ventricular myocardium. On the EKG, a PVC appears as a wide, bizarre-shaped QRS complex with no preceding P wave. Many times the QRS complex points in the opposite direction from the patient's normal QRS complexes. Also, the T wave that follows is wider and larger and usually points in the opposite direction from the QRS complex (see EKG strips on next two pages). What happens? The ventricles are stimulated prematurely (right after their repolarization phase) and contract before the expected time.

The ventricular depolarization-repolarization cycle consists of five periods: the normal excitable period, the absolute refractory period, the relative refractory period, the vulnerable period, and the supernormal period.

The cycle begins (the normal excitable period) when the impulse reaches the bundle of His, causing ventricular depolarization to begin and ventricular contraction to take place.

After the contraction, a short period of relaxation occurs in which the ventricles are resting, or repolarizing. The earliest stage of repolarization is the second phase, or absolute refractory period. During this phase, the cardiac cells are depleted of energy so they can't respond to any stimuli. On the EKG, this period begins during the QRS complex and lasts into the ST segment.

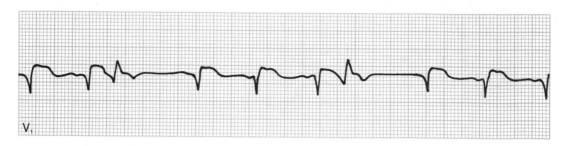

V₁

Unifocal PVCs

Note: The following information is the same for both unifocal PVCs (shown above) and multifocal PVCs (see opposite page).

EKG criteria:
- QRS complex is wide, bizarre, and distorted and usually deflects in opposite direction from patient's normal QRS complex.
- T wave of PVC deflects in opposite direction from QRS complex.
- P waves are not usually visible.
- Compensatory pause follows PVC.

Treatment
These drugs may be administered alone or in combination:
- Lidocaine, 50 to 100 mg, I.V., as a bolus followed by an I.V. of 2 g of lidocaine in 500 ml dextrose 5% in water to be infused at a rate of 1 to 4 mg/minute
- Procainamide (Pronestyl) I.V., 100 mg, I.V. push over 5 to 10 minutes followed by an I.V. of 1 g in 500 ml of dextrose 5% in water at 1 to 4 mg/min.
- Potassium chloride I.V.
- Quinidine by mouth
  Temporary pacemaker may need to be inserted.
  If PVC induced by digitalis, withhold dosage; if induced by hypoxia, give oxygen.
  Note: A malpositioned CVP line, pacing catheter, or pulmonary artery catheter may cause PVCs. Placement should be checked.

During the third, or relative refractory, period the cells can respond only to strong stimuli. This period extends from the remainder of the ST segment to the early part of the T wave.

The vulnerable period — the fourth phase — is the most delicate in the cycle. Some of the cells are fully repolarized, others partially repolarized. On the EKG, the vulnerable period occurs at the peak of the T wave. In any patient, particularly one who has organic heart disease, a single PVC occurring during this phase (R on T phenomenon) could initiate ventricular tachycardia or ventricular fibrillation.

Thus, the seriousness of PVCs is determined not only by how often they occur, but also by how close they are to the T wave of the preceding beat (coupling interval).

The fifth phase of the cycle, or supernormal period, occurs when repolarization is nearly completed; hence, the ventricles can respond to stimulation. This is when most PVCs occur. On the EKG, the supernormal period is at the end of the T wave.

If you suspect that the patient is having PVCs, check his rhythm strip for two things. First, see if each PVC occurs at exactly the same time after a normal beat. To do this, measure from the normal QRS complex to the PVC, and then check this interval for all the other premature beats. If all intervals are exactly the same, *fixed coupling* is occurring; that is, the interval between the normal and abnormal beats has not varied. To be sure coupling remains fixed, be alert to any changes in the interval.

Second, observe the pause after the PVC. Measure three consecutive QRS complexes. Then compare this interval with the interval occupied by the PVC and its preceding and succeeding QRS complexes. If the intervals are the same, or nearly so, the PVC has produced a *compensatory pause;* this means enough time was allowed after the PVC for the SA

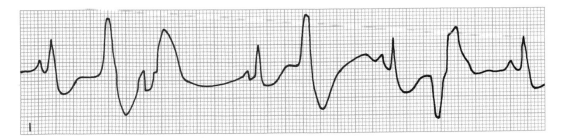

node to reset itself and resume normal conduction.

If the pause is less than compensatory, you should suspect that the premature beat is not a PVC but a premature atrial contraction (PAC) or a junctional premature beat. The QRS complexes of these dysrhythmias may resemble those of PVCs on the rhythm strip, but they generally don't have fixed coupling. If in doubt, suspect the worst.

PVCs may be *unifocal* or *multifocal*. All unifocal PVCs look alike because they originate in the same single ectopic focus (see opposite page). Multifocal PVCs, however, do not look alike — they change configuration and direction — because they originate from more than one irritable ectopic focus (shown above). Multifocal PVCs, often a sign of digitalis toxicity or severe myocardial disease, are the more dangerous.

In a few cases, a PVC will occur between two normal cycles. Called *interpolated PVCs,* they do not disturb the heart's basic sinus rhythm.

Another type of PVC is the *fusion beat,* which stimulates the ventricles at the same time that the normal stimulus occurs. Thus, on the rhythm strip, the QRS complex is wide, but it occurs at the expected time without a compensatory pause.

Parasystole, or pararhythm, is another type of PVC. In this dysrhythmia, the patient's own basic rhythm and a parasystole are functioning independently. The parasystolic focus discharges a regular stimulus, causing PVCs at any time in the cycle — as fusion beats, interpolated beats, and other random beats. Although the parasystole is perfectly regular, the coupling time *varies* with each PVC; therefore, a parasystole could occur during the vulnerable period, but rarely causes a run of ventricular tachycardia.

How PVCs are treated
Although isolated PVCs may require no treatment, those oc-

Multifocal PVCs
(For criteria and treatment see opposite page.)

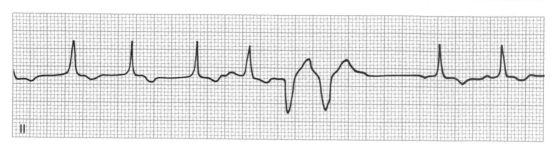

Michael's EKG (PVCs in pairs)

curring in clusters or salvos (groups of two, three, or five) do require treatment. So do frequent PVCs (more than 5 or 6/minute), multifocal PVCs, and couplets.

The primary aim of treatment is to quiet the irritable myocardium. This is best accomplished by administering a lidocaine bolus, followed by a continuous drip. But what if lidocaine is contraindicated, as in severe AV block or allergy? In many cases, procainamide will do just as well. Or quinidine may be given by mouth. Some doctors prefer a combination of drugs. Or in some cases, the only treatment required is good respiratory care (relieving hypoxia) or adding potassium chloride to an I.V.

PVCs tend to occur in patients with slow heart rates; hence, PVCs are often associated with poor cardiac output. Restoring adequate output can best be accomplished by inserting a temporary pacemaker if severe bradycardia or AV block are present.

A variety of measures may be used in a single case, as the following shows.

Michael C., age 45, was admitted to our CCU complaining of substernal pain. His admission EKG showed changes in leads V_1 and V_6. His ST segments were elevated, indicating a possible anterolateral myocardial infarction. He had a normal sinus rhythm with rare PVCs.

Two hours later, the PVCs were occurring at a rate of 5 to 6/minute, all unifocal. Our standing orders called for administering a bolus of lidocaine, 50 mg. The ventricular irritability subsided. However, 3 hours later the PVC's started again — this time in pairs (see above), and Michael was started on procainamide.

Whatever the treatment, your responsibilities in caring for patients with PVCs are as follows:

1. Determine whether the PVCs are unifocal or multifocal.

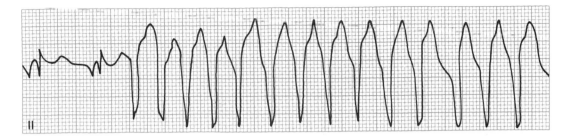

2. Check the location of the PVCs in respect to the T waves on the rhythm strip.

3. Observe the effects of the PVCs on the patient.

4. Be alert for runs of three or more PVCs (ventricular tachycardia).

5. Note any medications the patient has been taking, particularly those that might cause PVCs.

6. Know *when* to call the doctor and *what* to report.

7. Be certain that medication and equipment are ready for any treatment that may be needed.

8. Thus prepared, remain calm and confident in any eventuality.

9. Watch for signs of hypokalemia and digitalis toxicity.

Ventricular tachycardia

In many instances, ventricular tachycardia is precipitated by a PVC that occurs in the vulnerable period of the ventricular repolarization cycle (the R on T phenomenon). In ventricular tachycardia, the rate ranges from 50 (slow ventricular tachycardia) to 220 (rapid ventricular tachycardia). On the EKG, ventricular tachycardia can be identified by wide but uniform QRS complexes and a regular rhythm (shown above).

Since most patients can't tolerate high ventricular rates for long, they must be treated quickly. For short runs of tachycardia (5 to 6 beats/minute alternating with slow regular rhythm), lidocaine may suffice; but for sustained runs, a direct-current shock of 250 to 400 W/second is usually necessary. This should be followed by the administration of myocardial suppressant drugs, such as lidocaine or procainamide.

Ventricular flutter

Sometimes called coarse ventricular fibrillation, ventricular

Ventricular tachycardia
EKG criteria:
- Ventricular rate ranges from 150 to 220 beats/minute.
- QRS complex is wide and bizarre.
- RR intervals usually are regular, but a slight irregularity may occur.
- P waves are obscured by QRS complex.

Note: A group of three PVCs constitutes a short run of ventricular tachycardia.

Treatment
These drugs may be administered alone or in combination:
- Lidocaine (Xylocaine)
- Procainamide (Pronestyl)
- Quinidine

Temporary pacemaker may need to be inserted for slow rates with short runs of ventricular tachycardia.

Direct-current shock may need to be applied if patient is rapidly deteriorating.

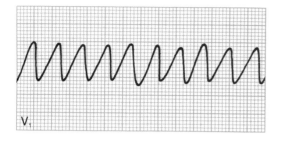

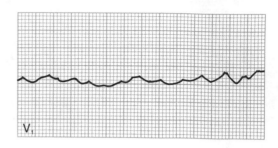

Ventricular flutter (above)
EKG criteria:
- Rapid, uniform, regular ventricular undulations may exceed 250/minute.
- QRS patterns are not distinct.

Treatment
- Direct-current shock may be applied, followed by lidocaine I.V. and sometimes quinidine or procainamide.
- If first direct-current shock is ineffective, should be repeated at 6-second intervals.
- Cardiopulmonary resuscitation should be given if direct-current shock fails.

Ventricular fibrillation (above right)
EKG criterion:
- Rapid, chaotic, ventricular rhythm lacks pattern.

Treatment
- Direct-current shock of 200 to 400 W/second should be administered immediatedly, followed by I.V. lidocaine or procainamide and cardiopulmonary resuscitation.

flutter often appears as a transient state between ventricular tachycardia and ventricular fibrillation. In fact, it may be so transient that it sweeps across the monitor screen before you can recognize it. On the rhythm strip, it appears as a clearly defined series of configurations that resemble the letter "m" (shown above left). The patient with ventricular flutter will show signs of poor cardiac output. He will collapse, may have a mild convulsive seizure, and may be incontinent.

If you're at a patient's bedside when he develops ventricular flutter, you might try a precordial thump with your closed fist. Usually, though, he'll need a direct-current shock of 200 to 400 W/second immediately. Until the defibrillator arrives, be sure to maintain his airway and circulation with CPR.

Ventricular fibrillation

Once you've seen this dysrhythmia, you'll never forget it. Ventricular fibrillation appears on the monitor as an uncoordinated, unrhythmic tracing with a pattern that resembles none of the dysrhythmias we've presented so far. The rhythm strip shown above right is an example. The patient will collapse, possibly with incontinence and tremors or seizures.

Minutes count. You must call for help immediately and begin treatment. The only effective treatment is direct-current shock of 200 to 400 W/second. One shock may be enough; if the first shock doesn't immediately reverse the dysrhythmia, another should be delivered within 6 seconds. Continue to aid in administering shocks and, if ineffective, initiate CPR. Also administer $NaHCO_3$ I.V., and if possible, obtain samples for blood gas analysis. Intubate the patient with an endotracheal tube and ventilate.

One person should prepare the medications the doctor may need — bicarbonate, vasopressors, lidocaine, epinephrine, and calcium gluconate. Have several intracardiac needles ready in

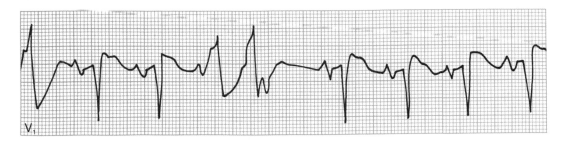

case they are needed.

Sometimes you can reverse ventricular fibrillation with a direct-current shock and drugs; sometimes you can't.

Alex's EKG

Guarded prognosis

While success in reversing ventricular fibrillation partly depends on how promptly you recognize the dysrhythmia and act, it also depends heavily on one factor you can't control: the condition of the patient's myocardium. Indeed, any ventricular dysrhythmia in a patient with a severely damaged myocardium implies a grave prognosis, as can be seen in the following case.

Alex, age 62, had had two previous infarctions before admission to our CCU. The initial diagnosis, possible lateral wall infarction, was based on a complaint of severe angina and an EKG that showed changes in the ST segment in leads V_5 and V_6.

Alex's admission EKG showed a moderately fast heart rate of 110, with occasional PVCs (less than 5/minute). Following standing orders for PVCs, we administered lidocaine drip, 4 mg/ml (2 g of lidocaine in 500 ml of dextrose 5% in water).

Soon after admission, Alex began to have more frequent PVCs (see EKG strip above). They were unifocal, but they came in pairs, which meant that Alex could quickly develop ventricular tachycardia and even ventricular fibrillation. We had no doubt that the ectopic beats were indeed PVCs and that they were not responding to lidocaine. So, we changed to procainamide, 1 g in 500 ml of dextrose 5% in water. Soon the PVCs disappeared, so we stopped the procainamide drip that evening and gave it orally.

Later that night, the PVCs recurred in pairs. Again we administered I.V. procainamide, but with no effect. We also administered propranolol. Still no effect. Yet, we detected no

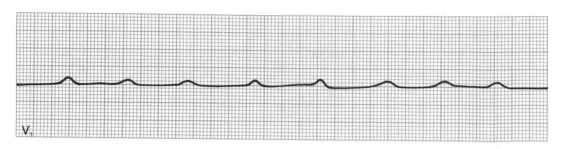

V_1

Asystole

EKG criteria:
- Either a straight line EKG or some chaotic incomprehensible imprint.
- P wave may be present but no ventricular contraction.

Treatment
- Sharp precordial thump
- CPR (immediate)
- Drugs:
    — Atropine I.V.
    — NaHCO₃ I.V.
    — Intracardiac epinephrine
    — Calcium gluconate I.V.
    — Vasopressors (Levophed, Aramine)
- Temporary pacemaker insertion

sign of congestive failure; his CVP was normal and his chest was clear.

Before long, the PVCs began occurring in groups of three to five (short runs of ventricular tachycardia). Again, we tried lidocaine — again no effect. Then Alex became hypotensive and he was deteriorating clinically. Before we could insert a temporary pacemaker, he had a short run of ventricular tachycardia, which quickly progressed to ventricular fibrillation. We aided in administering several direct-current shocks of 300 W/second but failed to resuscitate him. Alex's myocardium was just too badly damaged from his previous infarctions.

Asystole

Of all cardiac emergencies, asystole (cardiac arrest or ventricular standstill) strikes the most fear in nurses. And little wonder. It is always life-threatening. But that doesn't mean that it's always fatal. In fact, many patients, particularly young ones with no serious underlying medical problems, survive episodes of cardiac arrest. Whether they do depends on the condition of their myocardium, function of the pulmonary system, and the alertness and informed action of nurses and doctors.

Literally translated, asystole means the absence of contraction — the heart doesn't beat. So, it typically appears on a monitor as a straight line. But that isn't always the case; asystole also can appear as a chaotic imprint (shown above) showing some excitability of myocardium, which indicates end-stage ventricular fibrillation.

A common cause of asystole is hypoxia from impaired respiratory function. It also can arise from several other noncardiac problems — to name a few, respiratory impairment caused by anesthesia, drug overdose, hemorrhage, or anaphylactic reactions. If it occurs in a cardiac patient who is being

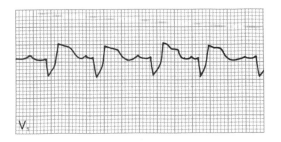
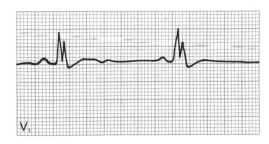

constantly monitored, it usually does so at the end stage of resuscitation or is preceded by marked, uncontrolled episodes of ventricular irritability.

Asystole is a true emergency. When it occurs, you must act quickly to initiate cardiopulmonary resuscitation. Start I.V. sodium bicarbonate and prepare an intracardiac injection of epinephrine for the doctor to administer when he arrives.

Bundle branch block

Conduction delays or blocks can occur in the bundle branches for the same reasons that they occur in the AV node or bundle of His. Although bundle branch blocks occasionally occur in healthy persons, they occur more commonly in patients with coronary artery disease or hypertension. Treatment is directed toward the associated heart disease rather than toward the block itself.

The heart actually has three bundle branches, because the left bundle branch divides into an anterior-superior division and a posterior-inferior division. The right bundle branch, however, is long and slender and doesn't divide until it reaches the endocardial surface of the right ventricle near the septum.

EKG changes resulting from bundle branch block are best seen in the precordial leads V_1 through V_6. Lead V_1 is the one we use to make the distinction between left and right bundle branch block, although with experience you will detect changes in the other leads as well.

Lead V_1 normally consists of a deep S wave preceded by a small wave. In right bundle branch block (shown above right), the R wave broadens or slurs and the QRS complex, which is now called RSR′, looks like an "M." Also, in right bundle branch block, the QRS complex is above the isoelectric line (a positive deflection).

In left bundle branch block (shown above left), the S wave

Right bundle block (above)
EKG criteria:
- QRS complex is prolonged to 0.12 second or more and is entirely above the isoelectric line in lead V_1.
- Right precordial lead (such as V_1 or V_2) shows RSR′ complex with ST depression and inverted T waves.

Treatment
- None may be needed.
- Treat underlying heart disease.

Left bundle block (above left)
EKG criteria:
- QRS complex is prolonged to 0.12 second or more and is below the isoelectric line in lead V_1.
- Deep S wave appears in V_1.

Treatment
- None may be needed.
- Treat underlying heart disease.

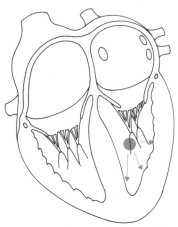

Pathway for ventricular dysrhythmias
Impulses for ventricular dysrhythmias bypass the atria altogether; instead, they come directly from single or multiple ectopic foci in the ventricles.

deepens and most of the QRS complex is below the isoelectric line (a negative deflection). In both left and right bundle branch block, the QRS duration is 0.12 second or more.

That the QRS complex is prolonged is readily understandable when we consider the mechanism of bundle branch block. Usually these blocks occur near the origin of the branch involved. When the impulse reaches the blocked area, it must find an alternate route to complete ventricular depolarization, or its conduction through the blocked area is delayed.

In right bundle branch block, conduction is normal through the left bundle branch and left ventricle. Because of the blocked right bundle branch, the right ventricle can be stimulated only by an impulse transmitted to it by way of the left ventricle. Conversely, in left bundle branch block, conduction is normal through the right bundle branch, so the left ventricle is stimulated by an impulse from the right ventricle.

Such detours cause delays in transmission of the impulse, which is reflected by a widening of the QRS complex. This widened QRS complex is the clue to bundle branch blocks.

A subclassification of complete bundle branch blocks is incomplete bundle branch block. Incomplete bundle branch block is more common than complete bundle branch block and shows all the abnormalities of a bundle branch block except that the QRS interval is 0.10 to 0.11 second. In most cases it occurs where a congenital defect or ventricular strain is present, such as with cor pulmonale and ventricular hypertrophy.

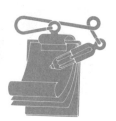

Remember these important points about ventricular dysrhythmias:
1. Identify PVCs by their wide, bizarre-shaped QRS complex, which lacks preceding P waves.
2. Determine PVC severity by how often they occur and how close they are to the T wave of the preceding beat.
3. Give lidocaine, as ordered, to treat short runs of ventricular tachycardia; aid in the administration of direct-current shock and follow with myocardial suppressant drugs, as ordered, to treat sustained ventricular tachycardia.
4. Know that success in reversing ventricular fibrillations depends on how quickly you recognize a dysrhythmia and act, as well as the condition of the patient's myocardium.
5. When asystole occurs, act quickly: initiate CPR, and administer direct-current shock, as instructed.

SKILLCHECK

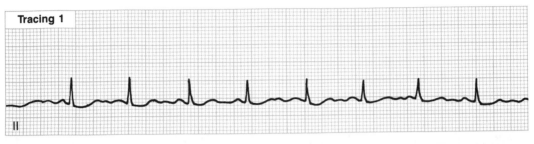

Tracing 1

II

Rate: Atrial _____   Ventricular _____
Rhythm: Atrial _____   Ventricular _____
Conduction: PR interval _____   QRS duration _____
Configuration/location: P wave _____   QRS complex _____
ST segment _____   T wave _____

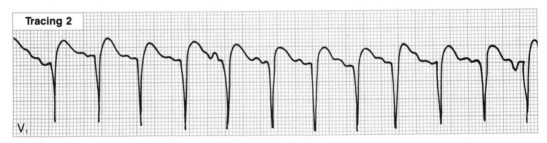

Tracing 2

V₁

Rate: Atrial _____   Ventricular _____
Rhythm: Atrial _____   Ventricular _____
Conduction: PR interval _____   QRS duration _____
Configuration/location: P wave _____   QRS complex _____
ST segment _____   T wave _____

(Answers on page 139)

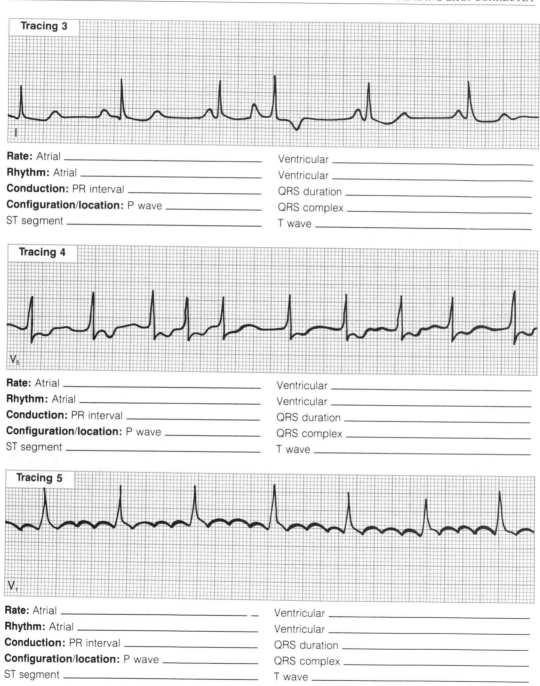

Tracing 3

Rate: Atrial _____ Ventricular _____
Rhythm: Atrial _____ Ventricular _____
Conduction: PR interval _____ QRS duration _____
Configuration/location: P wave _____ QRS complex _____
ST segment _____ T wave _____

Tracing 4

Rate: Atrial _____ Ventricular _____
Rhythm: Atrial _____ Ventricular _____
Conduction: PR interval _____ QRS duration _____
Configuration/location: P wave _____ QRS complex _____
ST segment _____ T wave _____

Tracing 5

Rate: Atrial _____ Ventricular _____
Rhythm: Atrial _____ Ventricular _____
Conduction: PR interval _____ QRS duration _____
Configuration/location: P wave _____ QRS complex _____
ST segment _____ T wave _____

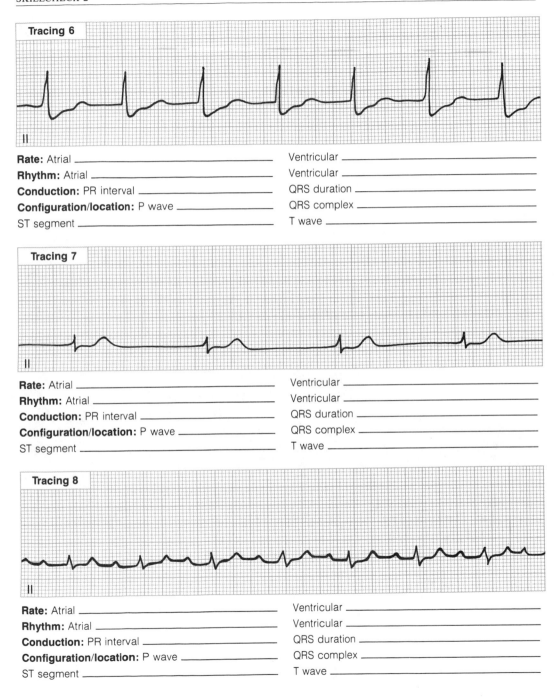

Tracing 6

II

Rate: Atrial _____   Ventricular _____
Rhythm: Atrial _____   Ventricular _____
Conduction: PR interval _____   QRS duration _____
Configuration/location: P wave _____   QRS complex _____
ST segment _____   T wave _____

Tracing 7

II

Rate: Atrial _____   Ventricular _____
Rhythm: Atrial _____   Ventricular _____
Conduction: PR interval _____   QRS duration _____
Configuration/location: P wave _____   QRS complex _____
ST segment _____   T wave _____

Tracing 8

II

Rate: Atrial _____   Ventricular _____
Rhythm: Atrial _____   Ventricular _____
Conduction: PR interval _____   QRS duration _____
Configuration/location: P wave _____   QRS complex _____
ST segment _____   T wave _____

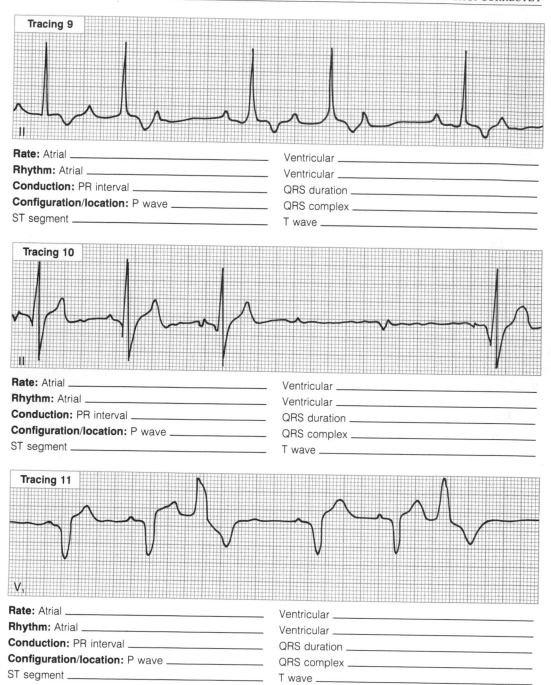

Tracing 9

II

Rate: Atrial _____   Ventricular _____

Rhythm: Atrial _____   Ventricular _____

Conduction: PR interval _____   QRS duration _____

Configuration/location: P wave _____   QRS complex _____

ST segment _____   T wave _____

Tracing 10

II

Rate: Atrial _____   Ventricular _____

Rhythm: Atrial _____   Ventricular _____

Conduction: PR interval _____   QRS duration _____

Configuration/location: P wave _____   QRS complex _____

ST segment _____   T wave _____

Tracing 11

V₁

Rate: Atrial _____   Ventricular _____

Rhythm: Atrial _____   Ventricular _____

Conduction: PR interval _____   QRS duration _____

Configuration/location: P wave _____   QRS complex _____

ST segment _____   T wave _____

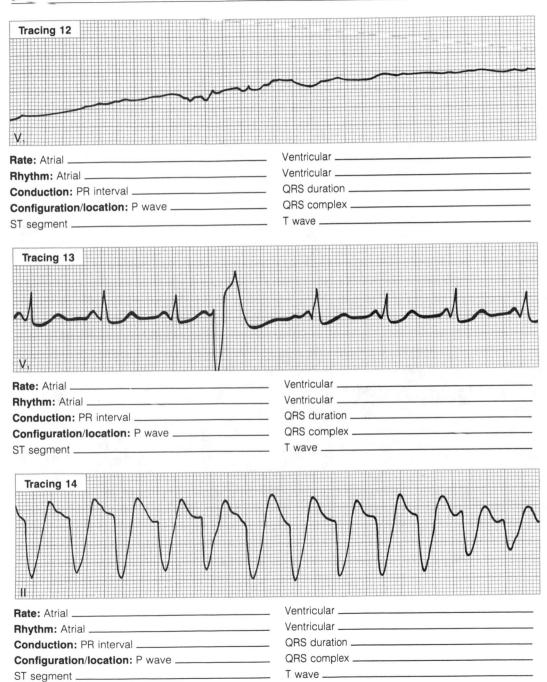

Tracing 12

V₁

Rate: Atrial _____   Ventricular _____
Rhythm: Atrial _____   Ventricular _____
Conduction: PR interval _____   QRS duration _____
Configuration/location: P wave _____   QRS complex _____
ST segment _____   T wave _____

Tracing 13

V₁

Rate: Atrial _____   Ventricular _____
Rhythm: Atrial _____   Ventricular _____
Conduction: PR interval _____   QRS duration _____
Configuration/location: P wave _____   QRS complex _____
ST segment _____   T wave _____

Tracing 14

II

Rate: Atrial _____   Ventricular _____
Rhythm: Atrial _____   Ventricular _____
Conduction: PR interval _____   QRS duration _____
Configuration/location: P wave _____   QRS complex _____
ST segment _____   T wave _____

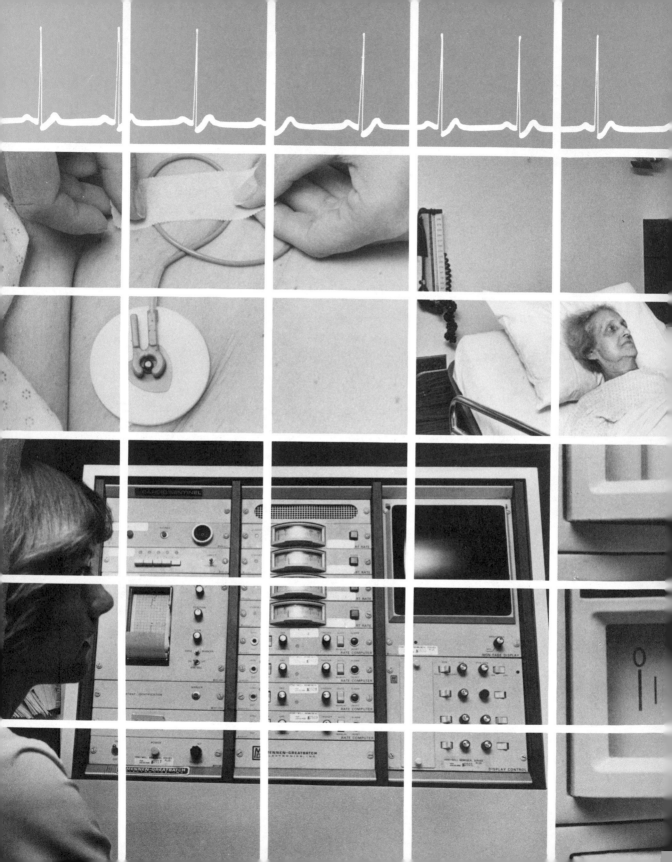

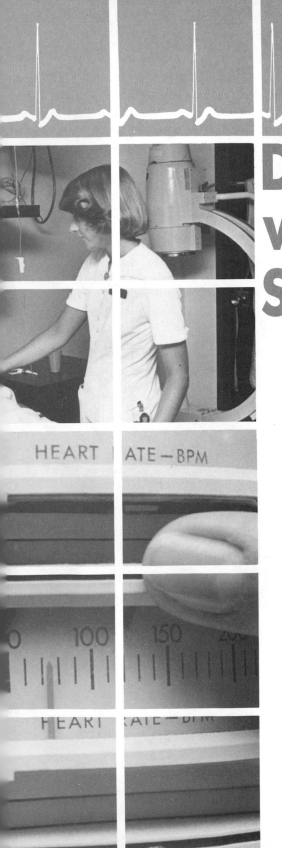

Dealing
with Special
Situations

Which uncommon EKG dysrhythmia, with QRS complexes that look like bundle branch blocks, causes frequent bouts of paroxysmal tachycardia?

What is the first EKG change you'll see in a patient with an acute MI?

If your patient has hypokalemia, what dangerous dysrhythmias will you find on his EKG tracing?

What nursing actions can you take to avoid a false-low rate during your patient's EKG?

If your patient repositions himself during an EKG, what should you expect to see on the tracing?

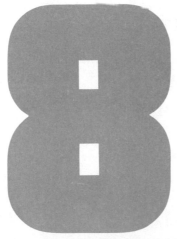

Uncommon EKGs:
When all else fails

In the past five chapters, we've presented the dysrhythmias you're most likely to see in your everyday practice. If you become thoroughly familiar with them, you'll be able to accurately interpret almost every EKG you may encounter. Still, others do exist. Even though they are highly uncommon, you should be aware of their names, salient features, and usual treatment.

The sample strips on the next few pages, and the information that accompanies them, should give you an adequate briefing on these uncommon dysrhythmias. Check a tracing for these dysrhythmias *only* when you have exhausted all other possibilities.

SA block
SA block is any block that prevents an impulse from the SA node from reaching the atria. Because of the interference with impulse transmission, the atria or ventricles do not contract. So, a cardiac cycle is missing on the EKG (see EKG strip on next page). Rhythm remains normal, though. That is, if you measure the tracing you'll find that the distance between QRS complexes before and after the dropped beat is *exactly* twice

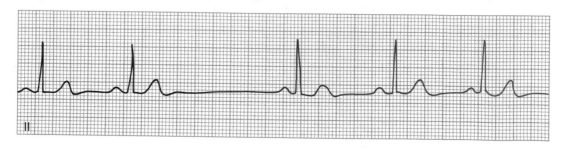

SA block

EKG criteria:
- Normal sinus rhythm with periodic pauses where an entire cardiac cycle (P, QRS, T) is dropped.
- Dropped cycle doesn't interfere with the normal rhythm; the interval of the dropped beat equals a normal cycle.

Treatment
- Usually none. Determine cause.

as long as normal. (This feature distinguishes SA block from sinus arrest.)

SA block can be caused by excess digitalis or quinidine, vagal stimulation (for example, carotid massage), or organic heart disease in the area of the SA node.

Blocked PAC

A blocked PAC (see top EKG strip on opposite page) is a premature impulse arising from an ectopic atrial focus that doesn't reach the ventricles. Cardiologists theorize that the PACs aren't conducted because of the AV node's refractory nature.

In a blocked PAC, a P wave (often abnormal in configuration) occurs without a QRS complex following it, much like an SA block. Unlike SA block, though, the rhythm is disturbed; the interval between QRS complexes is *longer or shorter* than two normal QRS intervals.

Wolff-Parkinson-White (WPW) syndrome

WPW, or accelerated conduction, most frequently occurs in men under 30. In it, impulses from the SA node can penetrate the AV node as they normally would or they can bypass the AV node and reach the ventricles directly through bypass tracts thought to be congenital, resulting in a short or absent PR interval.

Because of the accelerated conduction, patients in WPW are prone to rapid heart rates. When their EKG strips have QRS complexes that look like bundle branch blocks, suspect WPW — especially in any patient with frequent bouts of supraventricular tachycardia or paroxysmal tachycardia. The middle rhythm strip on the opposite page shows a classic example of WPW and illustrates the WPW syndrome. In true WPW, however, the EKG would also show runs of paroxys-

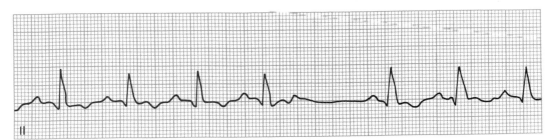

II

Blocked PAC

EKG criteria:
- P wave occurs early and is often of a different configuration and direction than normal P wave.
- No QRS complex follows pre-mature P wave.
- Interval with dropped QRS is less than a normal cycle.

Treatment
- If numerous blocked PACs occur, consider hypokalemia and check for digitalis or ischemia toxicity.
- Administer digitalis, quinidine, or beta blockers, as ordered.

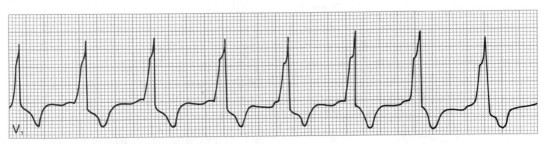

V₁

Wolff-Parkinson-White (WPW) syndrome

EKG criteria:
- PR interval is very short (less than 0.10 second).
- QRS complex is wide (0.11 to 0.14 second) or slurred (looks like bundle branch block).
- Delta waves are present at upstroke of QRS complex.
- Tracing shows runs of paroxysmal tachycardia, which appear as ventricular tachycardia.

Treatment
- Quinidine or procainamide sometimes effective; lidocaine I.V. for wide complex tachycardia.
- Ligation of AV node and permanent bipolar pacemaker.
- Cardioversion.

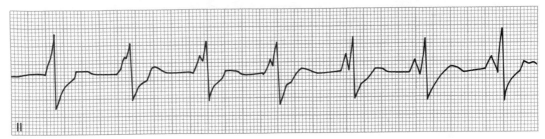

II

AV dissociation

EKG criteria:
- QRS complex is normal.
- Atrial rate and ventricular rate are different (no relationship between P waves and QRS complex); ventricular rate is higher.
- PR interval varies or is absent.

Treatment
- If caused by digitalis toxicity, discontinue drug.

mal supraventricular tachycardia.

AV dissociation

When the atria and ventricles are controlled by two different pacemakers due to impaired conduction through the AV node, the condition is known as AV dissociation. In this condition, the SA node paces the atria and the AV node paces the ventricles. The ventricular rate therefore is higher than the atrial rate, causing junctional tachycardia. AV dissociation is often caused by digitalis toxicity. In almost every case, it is a transient dysrhythmia.

On an EKG, AV dissociation produces varying atrial and ventricular rates, and may or may not produce a normal QRS complex (see bottom EKG strip on previous page). Because the P waves are unrelated to the QRS complexes, PR intervals will vary or may even be absent.

Note: Complete heart block equals AV diseases but not all AV disease equals complete heart block.

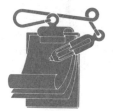

Remember these important points about uncommon EKGs:
1. On a rhythm strip showing an SA block, be aware that the distance between QRS complexes before and after the dropped beat is twice as long as normal.
2. Consider the following as possible causes of SA block: digitalis or quinidine toxicity, vagal stimulation, or organic heart disease in the SA node area.
3. Watch for WPW in any patient who experiences frequent bouts of paroxysmal tachycardia with QRS complexes that look like bundle branch blocks.
4. Suspect a blocked PAC when a P wave occurs without a QRS complex following it.
5. On a rhythm strip, be aware that AV dissociation produces varying atrial and ventricular rates, and may or may not produce a normal QRS complex.

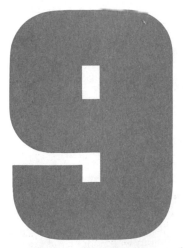

Two life-threatening conditions:
An insight

An EKG can be invaluable in diagnosing dysrhythmias. But it also can be invaluable in diagnosing several conditions that can precipitate dysrhythmias — specifically, congenital heart disease, pericarditis, pericardial effusion, electrolyte imbalance, and myocardial infarction.

I'm sure you've cared for at least one patient with one of these life-threatening conditions. Take a minute and pick one of your patients and think about his case history. Was an EKG one of the clues used to diagnose his condition? If not, why?

In some cases, your patient's condition may have been discovered through other means — through lab tests for electrolyte imbalance or through observation and the patient's medical history for myocardial infarction or pericarditis. Remember that the EKG changes can't give you quantitative results. So think of EKG changes as a clue to your patient's condition. In the next few pages, you'll learn which specific EKG changes to look for.

Detecting potassium imbalances
Both calcium and potassium play an important role in cardiac rhythm. For the most part, though, EKG interpretation has

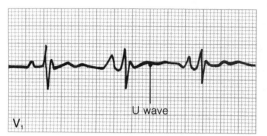

Signs of hypokalemia

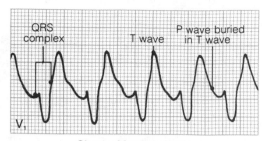

Signs of hyperkalemia

only limited value in detecting calcium imbalances since the EKG changes are almost imperceptible: a slightly shortened QT segment in hypercalcemia and a lengthened QT segment in hypocalcemia.

But, with potassium imbalance, the EKG changes can be a useful diagnostic tool.

Potassium imbalance affects the electrical activity of muscle, including the myocardium. At a normal serum level of 3.5 to 5.0 mEq/liter, potassium helps maintain normal cardiac rhythm. But an excess or deficit of potassium can cause dangerous dysrhythmias.

If mild, *hypokalemia* (low serum potassium levels) may cause only muscular weakness and fatigue. The myocardial effects include atrial or ventricular irritability. But, if severe, it can cause severe muscle weakness, paralysis, atrial tachycardia with varying degrees of block, and ventricular premature beats that may progress to ventricular tachycardia and fibrillation. These dangerous dysrhythmias are particularly apt to occur in patients on diuretics that can cause potassium depletion. With hypokalemia, digitalis toxicity can readily occur.

Early signs of hypokalemia are prominent U waves, a prolonged QT interval, and flat or inverted T waves (see above left). Usually the T waves will not flatten or invert until potassium depletion reaches a severe stage. A false impression of a prolonged QT interval may occur when the U wave is mistaken for the T wave.

Though less common, severe *hyperkalemia* (high serum potassium level) also can be highly dangerous since it can prevent the heart from conducting its electrical impulses. This can cause paroxysmal tachycardia, premature contractions, atrial flutter, atrial fibrillation, or cardiac arrest. Cardiac arrest is usually preceded by loss of P waves; widened QRS complexes;

and eventually, ventricular tachycardia, ventricular fibrillation, or standstill.

Early signs of hyperkalemia are small P waves, a widened QRS complex, and especially tall, tent-shaped T waves (see EKG strip at top right on previous page). These changes relate almost precisely to specific serum potassium levels: usually changes in the T waves indicate a level of 6.0 to 7.0 mEq/liter, and widening of the QRS complex indicates a level of 8.0 to 9.0 mEq/liter (a level that can quickly result in death).

EKGs and MIs
Unfortunately, EKGs won't always help you recognize myocardial infarction (MI). Some patients may not develop any EKG changes for several days, when they begin to show up only on serial tracings. And others with abnormally shaped chests or abnormal EKG patterns to begin with (for example, from prior infarctions) may never show characteristic EKG changes indicating an acute MI. Sometimes, too, the EKG changes may be so transient that you'll miss them on routine tracings. Or the EKG may not detect an infarct if it's small. In such cases, you'll have to rely solely on your observation of the patient, your knowledge of his medical history, and his physical exam.

But, with some MI patients, the EKG can be a valuable supplement to your observations. Let's begin by reviewing the pathologic changes that an MI causes and how these changes affect the EKG.

The most common cause of acute myocardial infarction is occlusion of a coronary artery, interfering with coronary blood flow to the myocardium. To visualize how obstruction of the blood flow can cause tissue damage and EKG changes, you should have some idea of the circulation to the myocardium (see illustration next page). Depending on the degree of oxygen deprivation caused by an obstruction, various tissue changes can result: an inner zone of tissue necrosis (the true infarct), a surrounding zone of severe injury, and an outer zone of ischemia (see illustration on page 93).

When these tissue changes occur, you'll note corresponding changes in your patient's EKG waveform. A flattened or inverted T wave reflects ischemia, a displaced ST segment indicates zone-of-injury, and a pathologic Q wave indicates necrosis. For Q waves to be abnormal, they should be larger

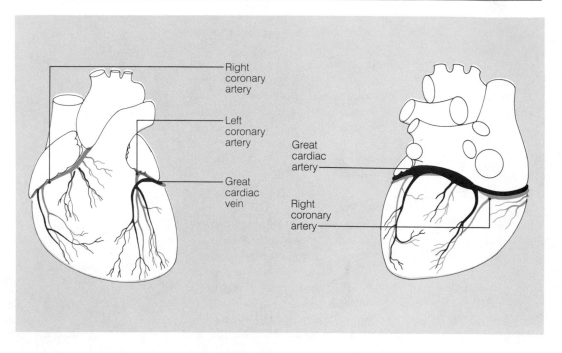

Coronary artery circulation

than one small square on the EKG paper horizontally (0.04 second) and vertically (0.1 mV). Q waves exceeding these dimensions are pathologic and usually indicate areas of infarction.

Q waves may appear immediately or within the first several days after the onset of symptoms. These Q waves will remain and usually can be detected for several years after the infarction has healed.

On the other hand, elevated ST segments will appear immediately but will return to normal from 1 to 4 weeks after the infarction. Because elevation of the ST segment is transient, it may be missed on the first EKG if the patient delays reporting his symptoms to the doctor. The T waves will become deeply and symmetrically inverted from 6 to 24 hours after the infarction and may return to normal from 2 weeks to several years later.

By coupling your knowledge about evolving EKG changes with your understanding of the leads and which areas of damage they detect, in many cases you can determine the extent and location of cardiac damage from your patient's EKG waveform.

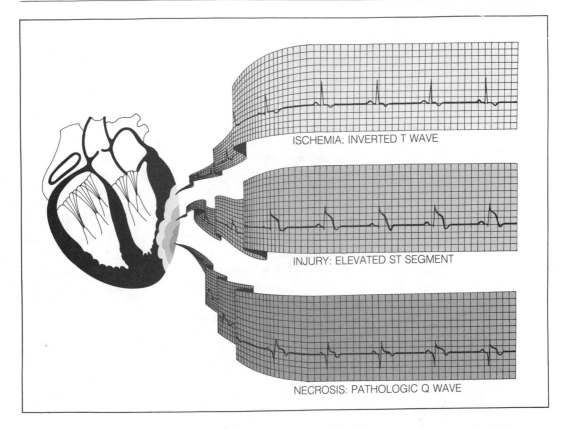

ISCHEMIA: INVERTED T WAVE

INJURY: ELEVATED ST SEGMENT

NECROSIS: PATHOLOGIC Q WAVE

Learning the leads

To assess the EKG of a patient who's had an MI, you must first assume that the patient's heart is in the normal position and that his chest is a normal shape. Then, you can localize the area of damage by picturing the areas of electrical activity that each lead records.

The precordial leads (V_1 to V_6) face the anterior and lateral aspects of the heart. Consequently, they can give you the best views of damage in those areas.

Leads V_1 and V_2, on the anterior chest at the fourth intercostal space to the right and left of the sternum respectively, lie just over the anterior surface of the right ventricle. So, changes in leads V_1 or V_2 indicate damage in that area, caused by an occlusion in the right coronary artery.

Lead V_3, between the fourth and fifth intercostal spaces and to the left of the septum, lies just over the ventricular septum.

EKG changes in an MI
The three pathologic changes that occur during an MI and their characteristic EKG changes are illustrated above.

It records activity of the septum and both the left and right ventricles. Changes in V_3 indicate damage in the septum or in the anterior wall of the left or right ventricle. Such damage is caused by occlusion of the branches of the left anterior descending coronary artery. To decide exactly which of these areas is damaged, you'd have to examine leads V_1, V_2, and V_4 as well.

Lead V_4, placed in the fifth intercostal space, lies over the septum and anterior wall of the left ventricle. When used with V_3, V_5, or V_6, it can pinpoint left ventricular damage in either the septum or anterior wall of the left ventricle, also caused by occlusion of the branches of the left anterior descending coronary artery.

Lead V_5 faces the lateral aspect of the left ventricle, while lead V_6 faces both the lateral and slightly posterior segments of the left ventricle. Changes in V_5 and V_6 are most apt to indicate damage to the left ventricle's lateral wall, caused by occlusion of the branches of the left circumflex coronary artery or distal left anterior descending coronary artery.

Lead aVL, which views the heart from the left shoulder, also can help pinpoint damage to the lateral wall of the heart when studied with leads I and V_6.

Of all the standard and augmented leads, aVR has the least diagnostic value. Since it faces the heart from the right shoulder, it records electrical activity in only a small portion of the right base of the heart. Except in rare cases, it isn't used for definitive diagnostic purposes.

Leads II, III, and aVF, however, record the electrical activity in the diaphragmatic (inferior) area of the heart. Therefore, EKG changes in these leads indicate inferior wall damage, usually from obstruction of the right coronary artery causing an inferior wall infarction. However, in 10% to 15% of patients, damage results from an obstruction of the circumflex artery.

In contrast, changes in leads I, aVL, and V_2 to V_5 indicate damage to the anterior left ventricle (anterior wall or anteroseptal infarction), caused by obstruction of the left anterior descending branch of the left coronary artery.

Finally, changes in leads I, aVL, and V_4 to V_6 indicate lateral wall damage (lateral wall infarction) most likely caused by an obstruction of the circumflex branch of the left coronary artery. (Occasionally, though, this infarction may be caused

EKG changes with anterior and inferior infarctions

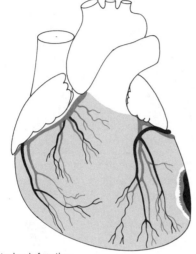

Anterior infarction

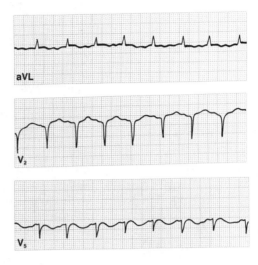

aVL

V₂

V₅

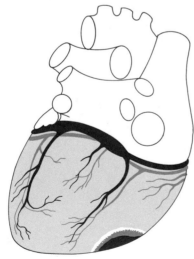

Inferior infarction

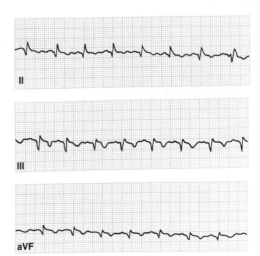

II

III

aVF

by an obstruction of the distal left anterior descending coronary artery.)

The illustrations on the previous page show the specific EKG changes you'll see with two common types of infarcts. Remember, though, that other conditions can produce EKG changes resembling those produced by acute myocardial infarction. For example, variant angina, pericarditis, acute pulmonary embolism, myocarditis, and left ventricular hypertrophy sometimes produce similar changes. And serial changes of a relatively small myocardial infarction may be so transient that they won't be detected by a routine EKG. In these instances, your evaluation of the patient's clinical course and laboratory data will help establish the specific diagnosis.

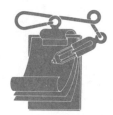

Remember these important points about detecting potassium imbalance and myocardial infarction on your patient's EKG:
1. Be aware that a potassium excess or deficit can cause dangerous dysrhythmias.
2. Be alert for early signs of hypokalemia: prominent U waves, a false impression of a prolonged QT interval, and flat or inverted T waves.
3. Consider small P waves, a widened QRS complex, and especially tall, tent-shaped T waves early signs of hyperkalemia.
4. If your patient's had an MI, observe his rhythm strip for an elevation in the ST segment, flattened and then inverted T waves, and pathologic Q waves.
5. Localize the area of damage on your patient with an MI by picturing the areas of the heart that each lead faces.

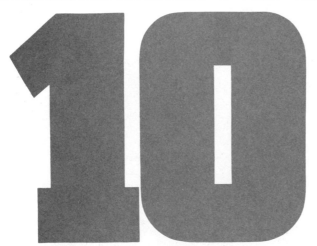

Cardiac monitors:
An overview

No discussion of EKG interpretation would be complete without some mention of cardiac monitors. Because, although they aren't the last word in EKG interpretation, they are a valuable diagnostic tool. Without them, all cardiac patients would be confined to bed so they could be constantly monitored by a bedside electrocardiograph. And, you'd spend most of your time running from one patient's room to the next, trying to keep up with the tracings coming out of several electrocardiographs.

Monitors allow patients mobility and give a quick reading on several patients at once. True, they have their limitations: greater risk of electrical interference, which can skew a reading, and the constant movement of the tracing, which doesn't allow you to measure EKG changes on the screen. But as early warning systems, monitors can be extremely useful. The trick is knowing how to operate them and how to detect mechanical errors in monitor tracings.

Monitor components
Although the many monitors on the market differ in design and operation, their basic components and function are similar.

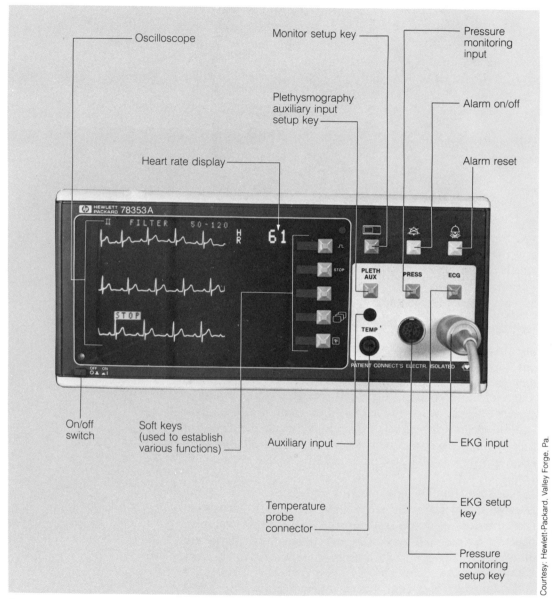

Oscilloscope

Monitor setup key

Pressure monitoring input

Plethysmography auxiliary input setup key

Alarm on/off

Heart rate display

Alarm reset

On/off switch

Soft keys (used to establish various functions)

Auxiliary input

Temperature probe connector

EKG input

EKG setup key

Pressure monitoring setup key

Courtesy: Hewlett-Packard. Valley Forge. Pa.

Top of the line

The sophisticated monitor shown above not only displays your patient's heart rate and lead II waveform, but also monitors body temperature and blood pressure. With proper pressure monitoring equipment, it has the capacity to indicate arterial blood pressure, aortic pressure, pulmonary artery pressure, central venous pressure, right or left atrial pressure, or intracranial pressure waveforms. You can also perform finger or ear plethysmography with this monitor.

The *oscilloscope* is the television-like screen on which the patient's electrocardiogram appears. As the heart beats, the tracing moves across the oscilloscope. If the monitor has a *freeze* button, the tracing can be temporarily held in one position for closer scrutiny.

Most monitors allow you to adjust the amplitude of complex on the oscilloscope. Remember, the complex must be large enough for the monitor to count the heart rate. To adjust amplitude, look for a gain knob or button marked amplitude. (In the monitor shown on the opposite page, the optimum amplitude is automatically set if the monitor is turned on before the patient is connected to it.)

The *heart rate* display shows the average number of cardiac cycles/minute and registers each cycle as an audible beep. (If you don't want a bedside monitor to disturb a patient, you can lower the volume of the beep with the *QRS loudness knob,* which may be located on the back of the monitor.) On some models, a *red flasher light* blinks every time a QRS complex appears on the oscilloscope.

The high– or low– heart-rate alarm setup is established by adjusting the appropriate button or slide tab. If you set the alarm system at the standard rates of 50 and 120, for example, any heartbeat falling below 50 or rising above 120 will trigger an audible alarm and in some models a printout.

If your monitor has a *lead selector,* it will allow you to choose which lead you want to monitor when more than three electrodes are used. If you notice a suspicious wave in one lead, it also will allow you to switch to another lead to double-check your suspicions.

Making the connection

Because monitors are highly sensitive machines, you have to take special care in setting them up and attaching them to patients. Where and how you apply them can make a big difference in the amount of information you get — or don't get — about your patient.

Before attaching the electrodes, plug in the monitor and turn it on. While it warms up, explain what you are going to do to your patient to allay his apprehension. Then select the sites for electrode placement (see page 101).

Wondering which leads are best for monitoring? The two most frequently used are the conventional method — tracing

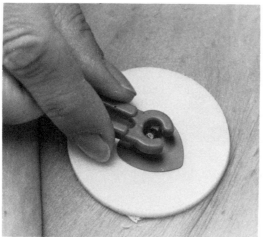

Attaching the lead wire

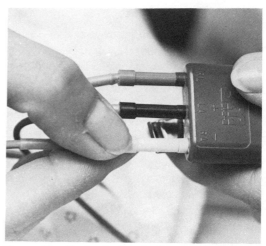

Connecting the lead wires to the receptacle

similar to lead II — and the modified chest lead (MCL$_1$) — tracing similar to V$_1$ of the full EKG. We'll describe the MCL$_1$ method here.

For an MCL$_1$, the positive electrode goes in the fourth intercostal space of the right sternal border, as for precordial V$_1$; the negative electrode in the clavicular hollow of the left shoulder; and the ground electrode in the clavicular hollow of the right shoulder.

After you've located these sites, prepare the patient's skin for electrode attachment. First shave 4" (10 cm) around each site (on male patients, if necessary), and cleanse with alcohol to remove skin oil. Allow to dry thoroughly. If the patient is perspiring, apply a commercial antiperspirant spray or tincture of benzoin.

Nearly all electrode disks come prepackaged and pregelled. After opening the disks, check them carefully for adequate gel. If the gel has dried on any of the disks, replace them. Apply all three disks on the designated sites, and make sure the adhesive forms a tight seal. Be sure to apply them in the clavicular hollows; applying them over muscles risks interference from muscle tremors and patient movement.

Next, snap the small electrode cables (lead wire — see photo above left) to the disks. Finally, insert the small electrode cables in the proper receptacles in the monitor cable (see photo above right). Be sure to insert the cable from the left

Three-electrode monitor

Lead II
Positive (+): Left side of chest, lowest palpable rib, midclavicular
Negative (−): Right shoulder, below clavicular hollow
Ground (G): Left shoulder, below clavicular hollow

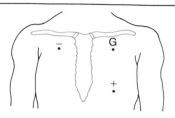

MCL₁

Positive (+): Right sternal border, lowest palpable rib
Negative (−): Left shoulder, below clavicular hollow
Ground (G): Right shoulder, below clavicular hollow

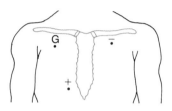

MCL₆
Positive (+): Left side of chest, lowest palpable rib, midclavicular
Negative (−): Left shoulder, below clavicular hollow
Ground (G): Right shoulder, below clavicular hollow

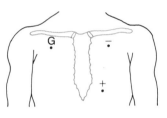

Five-electrode monitor

V₁ through V₆
Positive (+): Left side of. chest, just below lowest palpable rib
Negative (−): Right shoulder, midclavicular
Ground (G): Right side of chest, just below lowest palpable rib
Inactive (I): Left shoulder midclavicular
Chest V₁: Fourth intercostal space to right of sternum
Chest V₂: Fourth intercostal space to left of sternum
Chest V₃: Halfway between V₂ and V₄
Chest V₄: Fifth intercostal space, midclavicular, left side
Chest V₅: Halfway between V₄ and V₆
Chest V₆: Fifth intercostal space at midaxillary line

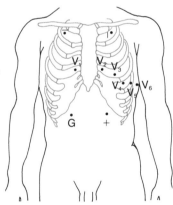

Guide to hardwire electrode placement

With five-electrode hardwire monitoring, as with a 12-lead EKG, you can record three standard limb leads (I, II, III), the three augmented limb leads (aVR, aVL, and aVF), and the six chest leads (V₁ through V₆) without distortion.

But suppose you're using a monitor with only three electrodes. You can establish the three standard limb leads and the three augmented limb leads without difficulty, because each arrangement requires only three electrodes. But you can't establish the V₁ through V₆ chest leads because they require five electrodes. So, when you have a three-electrode monitor, use the modified chest leads described in this chart instead. These leads require only three electrodes, but yield readings similar to the V₁ and V₆ chest leads. Modified chest leads are abbreviated as MCL₁ and MCL₆. You'll find that, for general monitoring on a three-electrode monitor, you'll probably use standard limb lead II, MCL₁, and MCL₆.

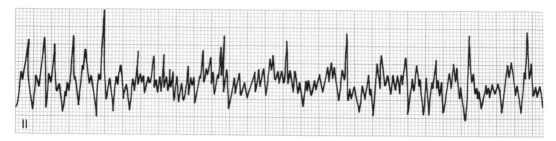

II

False–high-rate alarm (muscle artifacts)

electrode " − " (left clavicle) into the receptacle marked RA (right arm); the cable from the right electrode " + " (along the right sternal border) into the receptacle marked LA (left arm). As you can see, the position of the electrode cables is reversed compared with the conventional method. The cable from the ground electrode (right clavicle) is placed into the receptacle marked G.

Although MCL_1 is the best lead for standard monitoring, you may want further information from other leads. Leave the ground and negative electrodes in place and simply move the positive electrode to another position. For example, to monitor a modified precordial V_6 lead, move the positive electrode to the left fifth intercostal space at the midaxillary line.

If your patient is a likely candidate for dysrhythmias, such as bundle branch blocks or ectopic beats, you can attach several electrode disks at lead locations across his chest. Then, to quickly switch from one lead to another, just move the positive electrode cable from disk to disk. If your monitor has a lead selector, use it to obtain various lead tracings when more than three electrodes are in place.

After you've started monitoring, periodically check the condition of the electrode disks. If the disks cause itching or irritation, reposition them. If they become loose, reapply them. If they still won't stick, replace them.

Tips on troubleshooting

Even minor disturbances in the monitoring system — electrical interference, loose electrodes, and patient movement, for example — can create major interference with the EKG tracing. That is why you should learn to identify and quickly correct the most common monitor problems. Naturally, your first step whenever you notice an artifact should be to check the patient for medical causes. If his condition appears stable, check the

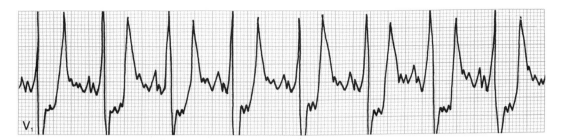

monitor for mechanical causes.

● *False–high-rate alarm.* As we've explained, the rate alarm averages the number of heartbeats/minute by counting the QRS complexes. But if a tracing contains tall waves from sources other than the heart, the monitor will probably record them as QRS complexes and falsely sound the high-rate alarm.

One possible cause of a false–high-rate alarm is skeletal muscle activity (muscle potential), which causes tall waves in a tracing (see EKG strip on previous page). To avoid this, apply electrodes away from large muscle masses, such as the pectoral muscles.

Another possible cause of a false–high-rate alarm is T waves as tall as, or taller than, the QRS complexes (see EKG strip above). Once you've ruled out hyperkalemia as the cause for abnormally high T waves, check for other problems with the monitor. Try repositioning the electrodes. If the T waves are still too tall, select a different lead — one where the QRS complexes have a higher amplitude than the T waves.

If the alarm persists, carefully check the system for loose electrodes, damaged or broken wires or cables, or improper cable connections. If these defects aren't causing the alarm, you may have set the alarm system too close to the patient's normal pulse rate. Reset the high-rate alarm slightly higher.

● *False–low-rate alarm.* If the contact between skin and electrodes is insufficient to transmit electrical impulses, a false–low rate will be recorded on the rate meter and sound the low-rate alarm. In some cases, the tracing may resemble idioventricular rhythm or it may resemble asystole. First, *check the patient*. If he doesn't seem to be in distress, check the electrodes. Chances are you'll find at least one electrode making poor contact with the skin.

A second possible cause of a false–low-rate alarm is patient movement. When a patient turns on his side, for instance, the

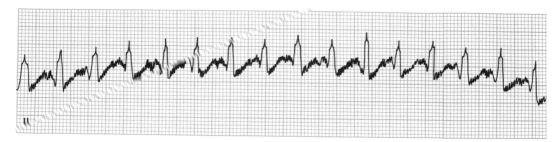

Electrical interference

axis of his heart shifts slightly, reducing the QRS amplitude. Since the rate meter can't detect the smaller QRS complexes, the low-rate alarm sounds.

If this happens, do not disturb the patient by asking him to change position; simply reset the gain knob to enlarge the QRS complexes.

If you're getting a baseline but no tracing, check the gain knob and the lead selector control to make sure they're positioned properly. If they are, check the cable connections. If the connections are firm, check the cables for damage and have a service technician check the monitor for defects.

Finally, check the low-rate setting on the pulse rate meter. The patient's heart rate may be too close to the low-rate setting. If so, increase the low-rate setting slightly, but be sure it's within a safe margin.

• *Electrical interference.* Interference caused by external electrical voltage (60-cycle alternating current) appears on the oscilloscope and rhythm strip as a widened baseline (shown above). Not only does electrical interference distort the EKG and obscure parts of the cardiac cycle, it can also pose an electrical hazard to the patient and staff.

Because the main source of electrical interference is improper grounding, ask the electrician to check the third prong in the power plug to make sure it's a true ground. Also move nearby electrical devices away from the monitor, if at all possible. If the patient is on an electrically operated bed, disconnect the bed's cable from the wall socket. In some cases, you can eliminate 60-cycle interference simply by replacing the electrodes.

• *Weak signals.* Indistinct or defective patterns on a monitor (see opposite page) may result from an improper gain-dial setting, from poor electrode contact with the skin, from improper small-electrode cable connection, or from monitor mal-

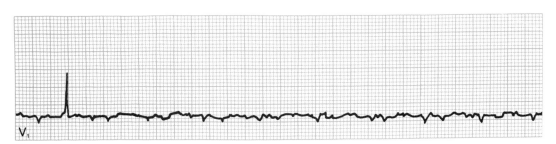

function. Without question, though, the most common causes are improper gain-dial setting and faulty contact between electrode and skin.

Weak signals

To correct weak signals, first try turning up the gain dial. If this doesn't improve the tracing, look for improper attachment of electrodes, too little or too much electrode jelly, and moist skin from perspiration. If these factors are causing the weak signals, reapply the electrodes.

• *Wandering baseline.* If electrode connections are inadequate, or if the electrodes move during patient movement or respiration, the monitor may register a wandering baseline (see next page).

When this occurs, first see if the patient's movement has disturbed the electrode connection. Then, check to make sure that tension on the cable isn't pulling the electrode away from the patient's body. Be sure the cable is secured to the patient's gown. If that's not the problem, look to see if the patient's respiratory movements are loosening the electrodes from his skin. If so, move those electrodes to another part of his chest — away from his ribs. If these checks fail to reveal the cause of the wandering baseline, assume that it's caused by external voltage variations; call the engineer.

Some final reminders
Cardiac monitors and electrocardiographs, through continuous surveillance, can give you priceless information. Not only can they help you assess dysrhythmias that need therapy, they can help you gauge the therapy's effectiveness.

But monitors and electrocardiographs cannot replace you, the skilled nurse. Only by deliberately and systematically checking clinical signs and symptoms and correlating them with your EKG findings can you truly assess a patient's condition. Remember that EKG interpretation is merely a tool.

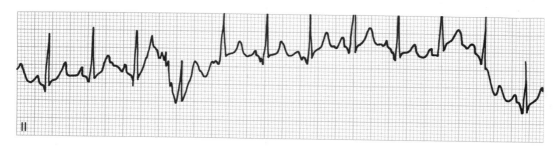

Wandering baseline

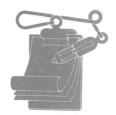

And like any tool, it's worthless unless you know how to use it correctly.

Remember these important points about cardiac monitors:
1. Know that the gain knob and amplitude help you regulate the size of the complex.
2. When using prepackaged, pregelled electrode disks, make sure the gel hasn't dried. If the gel has dried on any of the disks, replace them.
3. When using a modified chest lead (MCL_1), place the ground electrode on the right shoulder, the negative electrode on the left shoulder, and the positive electrode on the sternal border.
4. Consider skeletal muscle activity (muscle potential) one possible cause of a false–high-rate alarm.
5. Ensure adequate skin-electrode contact to avoid a false–low-rate alarm.

SKILLCHECK

Tracing 1(a)

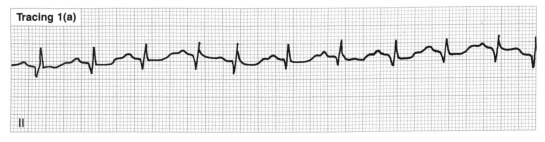

II

Tracing 1(b)

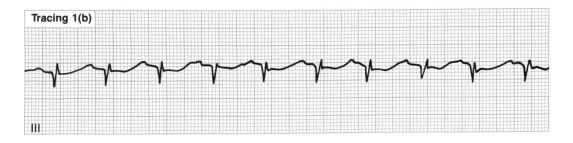

III

Tracing 1(c)

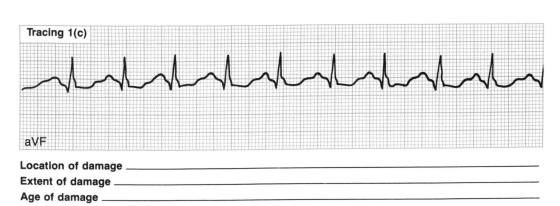

aVF

Location of damage _____

Extent of damage _____

Age of damage _____

(Answers on page 140)

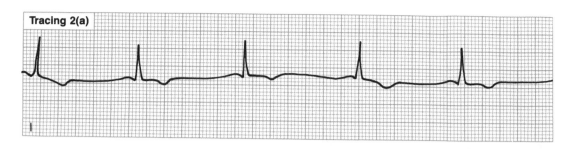

Tracing 2(a)

I

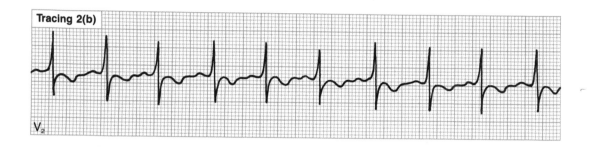

Tracing 2(b)

V₂

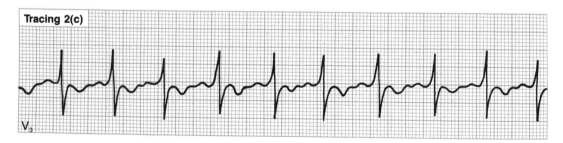

Tracing 2(c)

V₃

Location of damage _____

Extent of damage _____

Age of damage _____

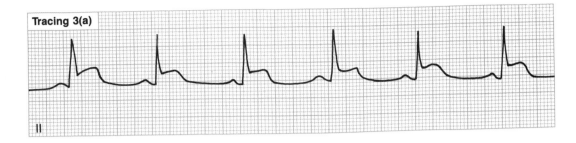

Tracing 3(a)

II

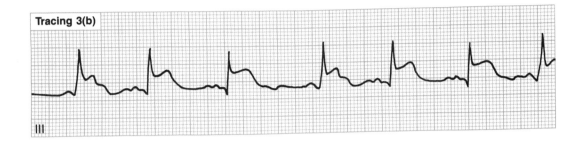

Tracing 3(b)

III

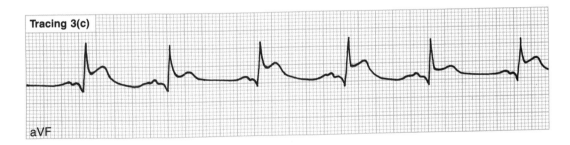

Tracing 3(c)

aVF

Location of damage _____

Extent of damage _____

Age of damage _____

The following tracings illustrate a few of the monitor problems discussed in Chapter 10. Try to diagnose each problem.

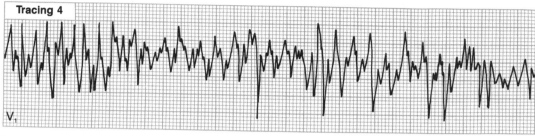

Problem _____

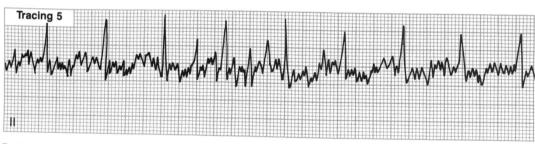

Problem _____

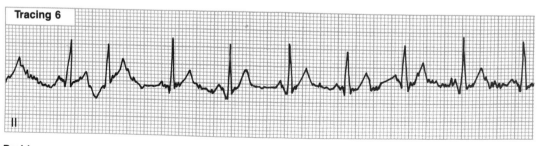

Problem _____

Tracing 7

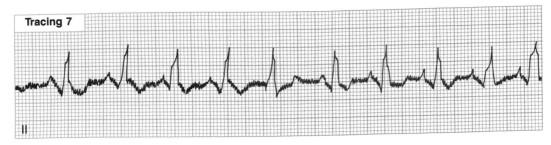

II

Problem _____

Tracing 8

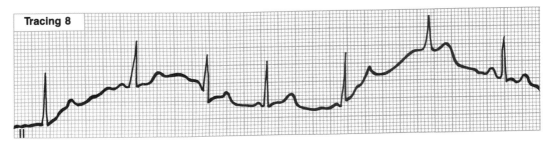

II

Problem _____

Test Yourself

Practice exercises to help sharpen
your EKG interpretation skills

If you've faithfully read the preceding chapters, carefully studied the sample tracings, and diligently worked the skillchecks at the end of each section, you should have a working knowledge of EKG interpretation. Now, you must perfect your interpretation skills. And the only way to do that is to practice, practice, practice.

On the following pages, you'll find numerous tracings that will give you an opportunity to do just that. As in real life, many have several answers. Be sure to study them carefully and record every finding.

As you go through these tracings, remember that they are self-tests — not a teacher's test. Our sole purpose in including them is to let you measure your progress and determine your strengths and weaknesses so *you* can decide where you need further study.

If one of your answers disagrees with the given answer, don't simply accept it as a mistake and go on to the next tracing. Instead, rework the tracing. Are your measurements accurate? Is the diagnosis consistent with those measurements? If your answer still disagrees with the given answer, reread the appropriate chapter and study the appropriate sample tracings. Are your measurements consistent with the criteria given for the sample tracings?

If, after scrutiny and research, your answer still seems correct and yet still disagrees with the given answer, you may have hit upon a tracing whose diagnosis is open to debate. Remember that EKG interpretation isn't an exact science. Even world-famous cardiologists have been known to disagree over the interpretation of some tracings, such as PACs and PNCs. The best you can do is to explore every possibility, to make sure your measurements are accurate, and to make the most logical, plausible interpretation.

After you've determined the correct diagnosis, we suggest you try to answer the key questions presented in Chapter 2: Where did the dysrhythmia originate? What is the heart doing? What treatment might be needed to correct the dysrhythmia, and what problems might that treatment create? What would happen to the patient if the dysrhythmia were not treated? What special nursing considerations are implied by this dysrhythmia? If you are unsure how to answer these questions for any specific dysrhythmia, reread the appropriate chapters and study the criteria and treatment information listed under the sample strips. Only by answering all of these questions can you get the full value from the self-tests.

One final word: This chapter is the end of the teaching portion of this book. But it should be only the beginning of your learning, because you must constantly practice the skills you've learned here if you want to become truly proficient at EKG interpretation.

A striking example of the benefits of practice is the experience of a young nurse who attended our EKG lecture series several years ago. After each session, she begged for more information and for additional rhythm strips to analyze. She read several books on EKG interpretation outside class and pestered our EKG technician for old tracings. Even after our lecture series ended, she continued interpreting every tracing she could get her hands on.

A year later, she transferred to the coronary care unit (CCU) at a larger teaching hospital. The chief cardiologist, after working with her for several weeks, commended her on her ability to analyze tracings, which compared favorably with that of most interns' and residents'. Even though she hadn't had any formal management training, he recommended her for promotion to head nurse in CCU. Her hard work, and lots of practice, paid off.

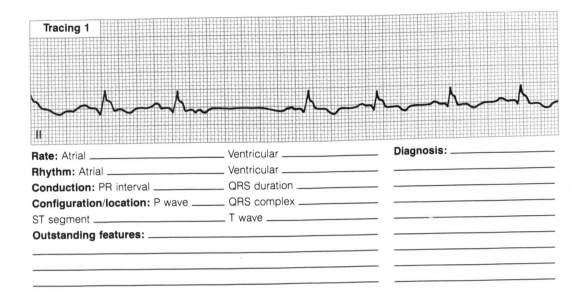

Rate: Atrial _____ Ventricular _____
Rhythm: Atrial _____ Ventricular _____
Conduction: PR interval _____ QRS duration _____
Configuration/location: P wave _____ QRS complex _____
ST segment _____ T wave _____
Outstanding features: _____

Diagnosis: _____

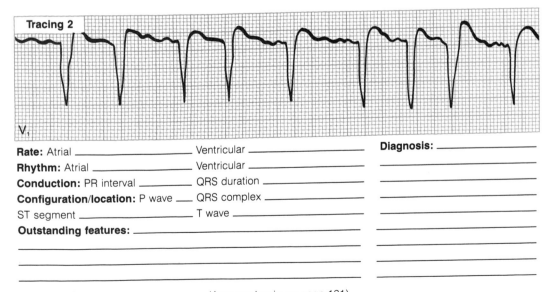

Rate: Atrial _____ Ventricular _____
Rhythm: Atrial _____ Ventricular _____
Conduction: PR interval _____ QRS duration _____
Configuration/location: P wave _____ QRS complex _____
ST segment _____ T wave _____
Outstanding features: _____

Diagnosis: _____

(Answers begin on page 131)

Tracing 3

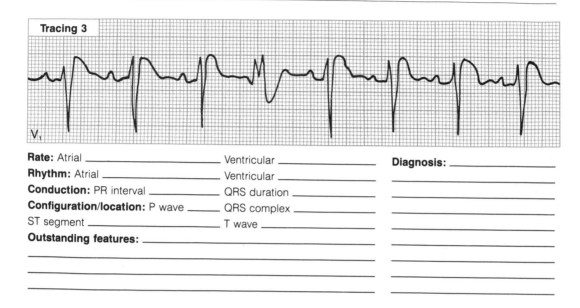

V₁

Rate: Atrial _____ Ventricular _____ **Diagnosis:** _____

Rhythm: Atrial _____ Ventricular _____ _____

Conduction: PR interval _____ QRS duration _____ _____

Configuration/location: P wave _____ QRS complex _____ _____

ST segment _____ T wave _____ _____

Outstanding features: _____ _____

_____ _____

_____ _____

_____ _____

Tracing 4

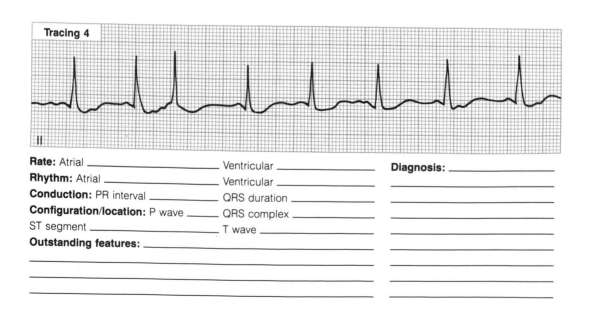

II

Rate: Atrial _____ Ventricular _____ **Diagnosis:** _____

Rhythm: Atrial _____ Ventricular _____ _____

Conduction: PR interval _____ QRS duration _____ _____

Configuration/location: P wave _____ QRS complex _____ _____

ST segment _____ T wave _____ _____

Outstanding features: _____ _____

_____ _____

_____ _____

_____ _____

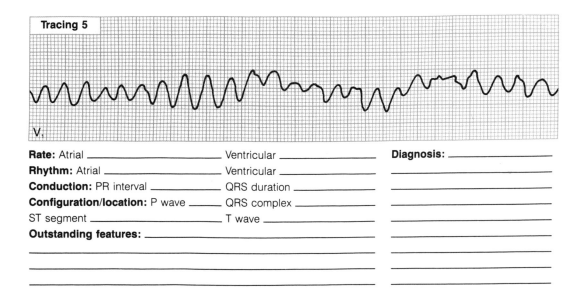

Tracing 5

Rate: Atrial _____ Ventricular _____ **Diagnosis:** _____

Rhythm: Atrial _____ Ventricular _____ _____

Conduction: PR interval _____ QRS duration _____ _____

Configuration/location: P wave _____ QRS complex _____ _____

ST segment _____ T wave _____ _____

Outstanding features: _____ _____

_____ _____

_____ _____

_____ _____

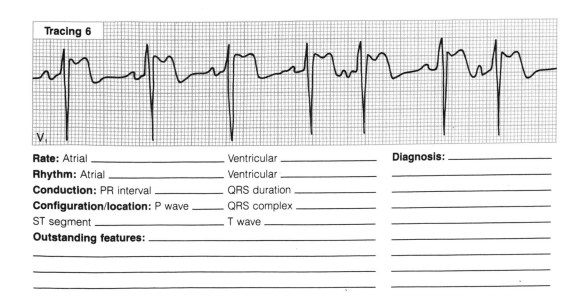

Tracing 6

Rate: Atrial _____ Ventricular _____ **Diagnosis:** _____

Rhythm: Atrial _____ Ventricular _____ _____

Conduction: PR interval _____ QRS duration _____ _____

Configuration/location: P wave _____ QRS complex _____ _____

ST segment _____ T wave _____ _____

Outstanding features: _____ _____

_____ _____

_____ _____

_____ _____

Tracing 7

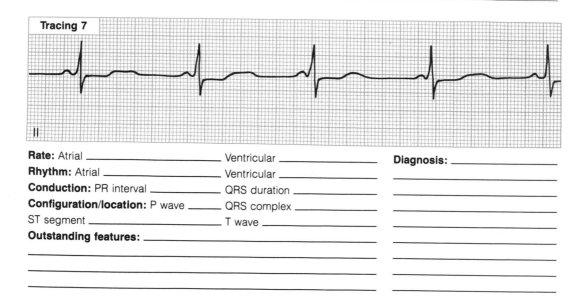

II

Rate: Atrial _____ Ventricular _____ **Diagnosis:** _____

Rhythm: Atrial _____ Ventricular _____ _____

Conduction: PR interval _____ QRS duration _____ _____

Configuration/location: P wave _____ QRS complex _____ _____

ST segment _____ T wave _____ _____

Outstanding features: _____ _____

_____ _____

_____ _____

_____ _____

Tracing 8

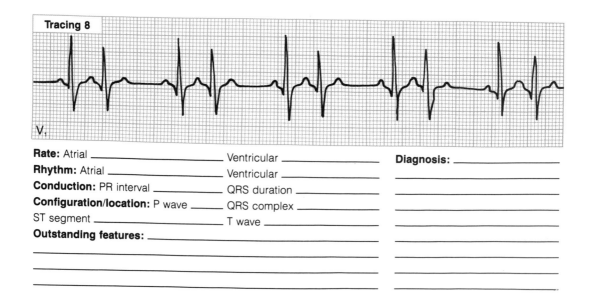

V₁

Rate: Atrial _____ Ventricular _____ **Diagnosis:** _____

Rhythm: Atrial _____ Ventricular _____ _____

Conduction: PR interval _____ QRS duration _____ _____

Configuration/location: P wave _____ QRS complex _____ _____

ST segment _____ T wave _____ _____

Outstanding features: _____ _____

_____ _____

_____ _____

_____ _____

Tracing 9

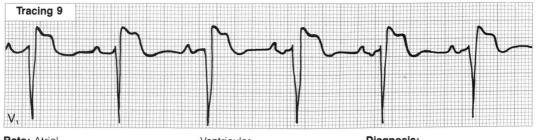

V₁

Rate: Atrial _____ Ventricular _____ **Diagnosis:** _____

Rhythm: Atrial _____ Ventricular _____ _____

Conduction: PR interval _____ QRS duration _____ _____

Configuration/location: P wave _____ QRS complex _____ _____

ST segment _____ T wave _____ _____

Outstanding features: _____ _____

_____ _____

_____ _____

_____ _____

Tracing 10

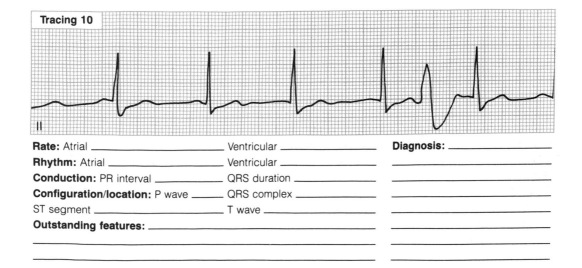

II

Rate: Atrial _____ Ventricular _____ **Diagnosis:** _____

Rhythm: Atrial _____ Ventricular _____ _____

Conduction: PR interval _____ QRS duration _____ _____

Configuration/location: P wave _____ QRS complex _____ _____

ST segment _____ T wave _____ _____

Outstanding features: _____ _____

_____ _____

_____ _____

_____ _____

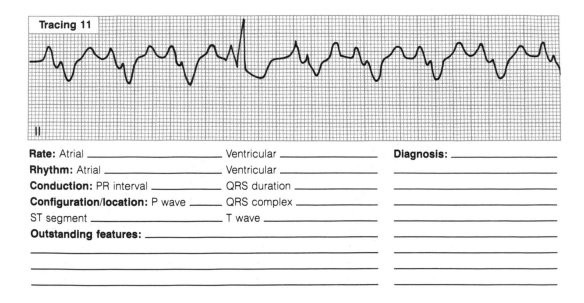

Tracing 11

II

Rate: Atrial _____ Ventricular _____ **Diagnosis:** _____

Rhythm: Atrial _____ Ventricular _____ _____

Conduction: PR interval _____ QRS duration _____ _____

Configuration/location: P wave _____ QRS complex _____ _____

ST segment _____ T wave _____ _____

Outstanding features: _____ _____

_____ _____

_____ _____

_____ _____

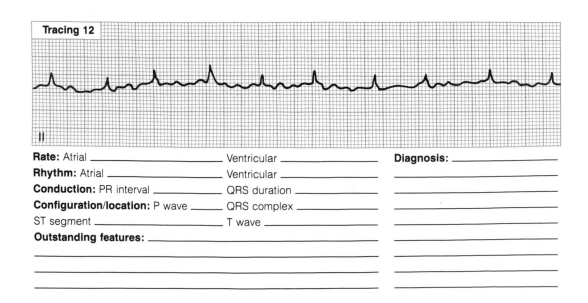

Tracing 12

II

Rate: Atrial _____ Ventricular _____ **Diagnosis:** _____

Rhythm: Atrial _____ Ventricular _____ _____

Conduction: PR interval _____ QRS duration _____ _____

Configuration/location: P wave _____ QRS complex _____ _____

ST segment _____ T wave _____ _____

Outstanding features: _____ _____

_____ _____

_____ _____

_____ _____

Tracing 13

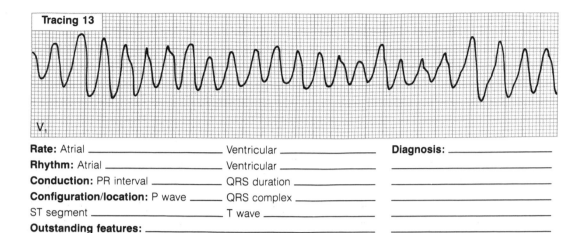

V₁

Rate: Atrial _____ Ventricular _____ **Diagnosis:** _____

Rhythm: Atrial _____ Ventricular _____ _____

Conduction: PR interval _____ QRS duration _____ _____

Configuration/location: P wave _____ QRS complex _____ _____

ST segment _____ T wave _____ _____

Outstanding features: _____

_____ _____

_____ _____

_____ _____

Tracing 14

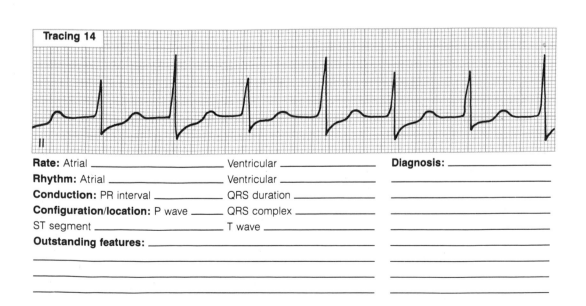

II

Rate: Atrial _____ Ventricular _____ **Diagnosis:** _____

Rhythm: Atrial _____ Ventricular _____ _____

Conduction: PR interval _____ QRS duration _____ _____

Configuration/location: P wave _____ QRS complex _____ _____

ST segment _____ T wave _____ _____

Outstanding features: _____

_____ _____

_____ _____

_____ _____

Tracing 15

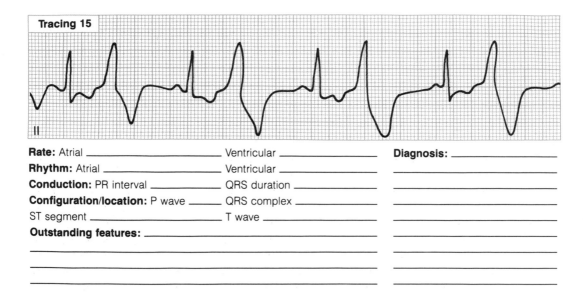

II

Rate: Atrial _____ Ventricular _____   **Diagnosis:** _____

Rhythm: Atrial _____ Ventricular _____   _____

Conduction: PR interval _____ QRS duration _____   _____

Configuration/location: P wave _____ QRS complex _____   _____

ST segment _____ T wave _____   _____

Outstanding features: _____

_____   _____

_____   _____

_____   _____

Tracing 16

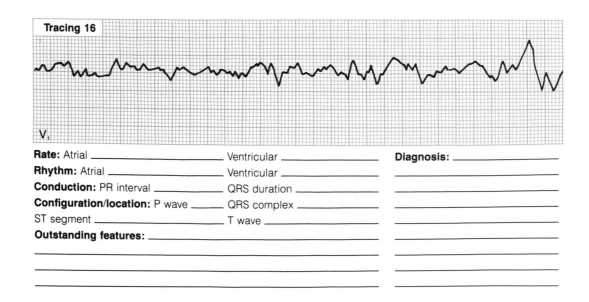

V₁

Rate: Atrial _____ Ventricular _____   **Diagnosis:** _____

Rhythm: Atrial _____ Ventricular _____   _____

Conduction: PR interval _____ QRS duration _____   _____

Configuration/location: P wave _____ QRS complex _____   _____

ST segment _____ T wave _____   _____

Outstanding features: _____

_____   _____

_____   _____

_____   _____

Tracing 17

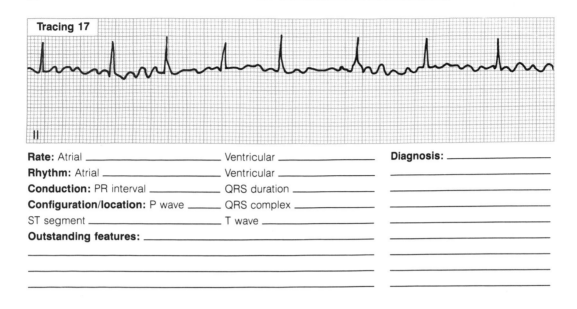

II

Rate: Atrial _____ Ventricular _____ **Diagnosis:** _____

Rhythm: Atrial _____ Ventricular _____ _____

Conduction: PR interval _____ QRS duration _____ _____

Configuration/location: P wave _____ QRS complex _____ _____

ST segment _____ T wave _____ _____

Outstanding features: _____ _____

_____ _____

_____ _____

_____ _____

Tracing 18

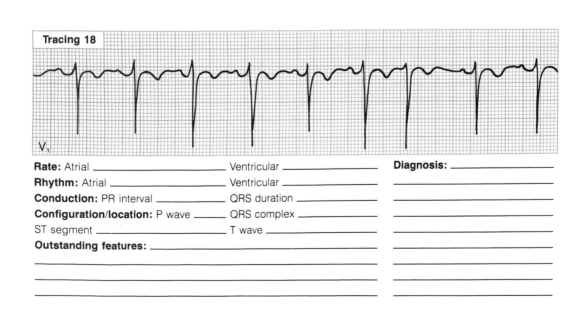

V₁

Rate: Atrial _____ Ventricular _____ **Diagnosis:** _____

Rhythm: Atrial _____ Ventricular _____ _____

Conduction: PR interval _____ QRS duration _____ _____

Configuration/location: P wave _____ QRS complex _____ _____

ST segment _____ T wave _____ _____

Outstanding features: _____ _____

_____ _____

_____ _____

_____ _____

Tracing 19

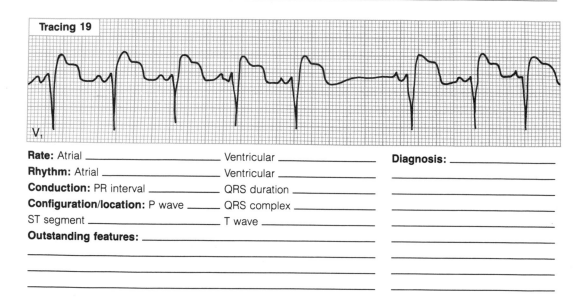

V₁

Rate: Atrial ＿＿＿＿＿＿＿＿＿ Ventricular ＿＿＿＿＿＿＿   **Diagnosis:** ＿＿＿＿＿＿＿

Rhythm: Atrial ＿＿＿＿＿＿＿ Ventricular ＿＿＿＿＿＿   ＿＿＿＿＿＿＿＿＿＿＿＿

Conduction: PR interval ＿＿＿＿＿ QRS duration ＿＿＿＿＿   ＿＿＿＿＿＿＿＿＿＿＿＿

Configuration/location: P wave ＿＿＿ QRS complex ＿＿＿＿   ＿＿＿＿＿＿＿＿＿＿＿＿

ST segment ＿＿＿＿＿＿＿＿＿ T wave ＿＿＿＿＿＿＿   ＿＿＿＿＿＿＿＿＿＿＿＿

Outstanding features: ＿＿＿＿＿＿＿＿＿＿＿＿＿＿＿   ＿＿＿＿＿＿＿＿＿＿＿＿

＿＿＿＿＿＿＿＿＿＿＿＿＿＿＿＿＿＿＿＿＿   ＿＿＿＿＿＿＿＿＿＿＿＿

＿＿＿＿＿＿＿＿＿＿＿＿＿＿＿＿＿＿＿＿＿   ＿＿＿＿＿＿＿＿＿＿＿＿

＿＿＿＿＿＿＿＿＿＿＿＿＿＿＿＿＿＿＿＿＿   ＿＿＿＿＿＿＿＿＿＿＿＿

Tracing 20

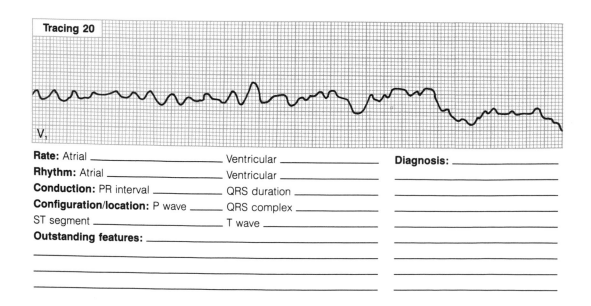

V₁

Rate: Atrial ＿＿＿＿＿＿＿＿＿ Ventricular ＿＿＿＿＿＿＿   **Diagnosis:** ＿＿＿＿＿＿＿

Rhythm: Atrial ＿＿＿＿＿＿＿ Ventricular ＿＿＿＿＿＿   ＿＿＿＿＿＿＿＿＿＿＿＿

Conduction: PR interval ＿＿＿＿＿ QRS duration ＿＿＿＿＿   ＿＿＿＿＿＿＿＿＿＿＿＿

Configuration/location: P wave ＿＿＿ QRS complex ＿＿＿＿   ＿＿＿＿＿＿＿＿＿＿＿＿

ST segment ＿＿＿＿＿＿＿＿＿ T wave ＿＿＿＿＿＿＿   ＿＿＿＿＿＿＿＿＿＿＿＿

Outstanding features: ＿＿＿＿＿＿＿＿＿＿＿＿＿＿＿   ＿＿＿＿＿＿＿＿＿＿＿＿

＿＿＿＿＿＿＿＿＿＿＿＿＿＿＿＿＿＿＿＿＿   ＿＿＿＿＿＿＿＿＿＿＿＿

＿＿＿＿＿＿＿＿＿＿＿＿＿＿＿＿＿＿＿＿＿   ＿＿＿＿＿＿＿＿＿＿＿＿

＿＿＿＿＿＿＿＿＿＿＿＿＿＿＿＿＿＿＿＿＿   ＿＿＿＿＿＿＿＿＿＿＿＿

Tracing 21

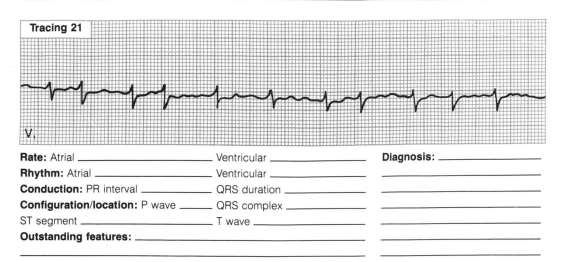

V₁

Rate: Atrial _____ Ventricular _____   **Diagnosis:** _____

Rhythm: Atrial _____ Ventricular _____   _____

Conduction: PR interval _____ QRS duration _____   _____

Configuration/location: P wave _____ QRS complex _____   _____

ST segment _____ T wave _____   _____

Outstanding features: _____   _____

_____   _____

_____   _____

_____   _____

Tracing 22

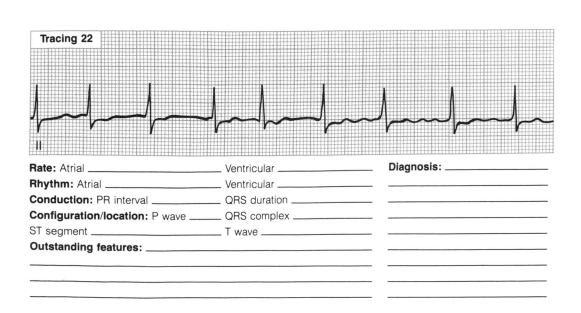

II

Rate: Atrial _____ Ventricular _____   **Diagnosis:** _____

Rhythm: Atrial _____ Ventricular _____   _____

Conduction: PR interval _____ QRS duration _____   _____

Configuration/location: P wave _____ QRS complex _____   _____

ST segment _____ T wave _____   _____

Outstanding features: _____   _____

_____   _____

_____   _____

_____   _____

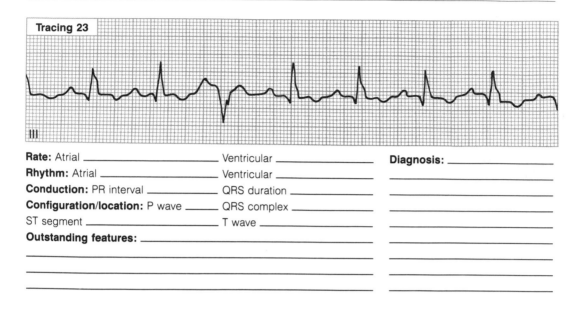

Tracing 23

III

Rate: Atrial _____ Ventricular _____ **Diagnosis:** _____

Rhythm: Atrial _____ Ventricular _____ _____

Conduction: PR interval _____ QRS duration _____ _____

Configuration/location: P wave _____ QRS complex _____ _____

ST segment _____ T wave _____ _____

Outstanding features: _____ _____

_____ _____

_____ _____

_____ _____

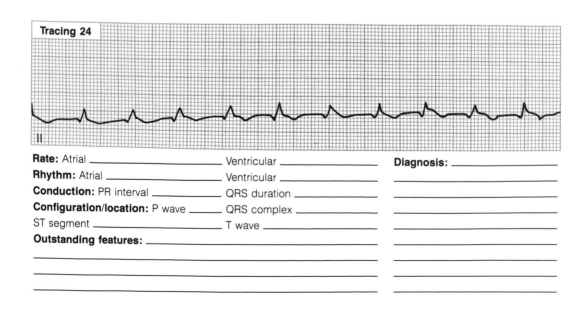

Tracing 24

II

Rate: Atrial _____ Ventricular _____ **Diagnosis:** _____

Rhythm: Atrial _____ Ventricular _____ _____

Conduction: PR interval _____ QRS duration _____ _____

Configuration/location: P wave _____ QRS complex _____ _____

ST segment _____ T wave _____ _____

Outstanding features: _____ _____

_____ _____

_____ _____

_____ _____

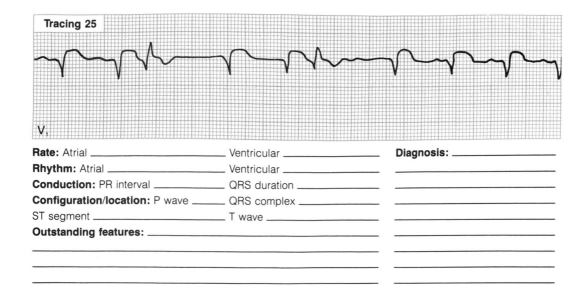

Rate: Atrial _____ Ventricular _____   **Diagnosis:** _____
Rhythm: Atrial _____ Ventricular _____   _____
Conduction: PR interval _____ QRS duration _____   _____
Configuration/location: P wave _____ QRS complex _____   _____
ST segment _____ T wave _____   _____
Outstanding features: _____   _____
_____   _____
_____   _____
_____

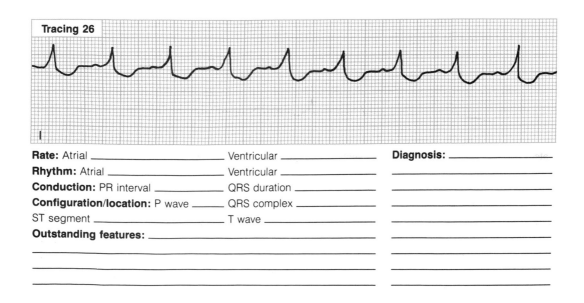

Rate: Atrial _____ Ventricular _____   **Diagnosis:** _____
Rhythm: Atrial _____ Ventricular _____   _____
Conduction: PR interval _____ QRS duration _____   _____
Configuration/location: P wave _____ QRS complex _____   _____
ST segment _____ T wave _____   _____
Outstanding features: _____   _____
_____   _____
_____   _____
_____

128

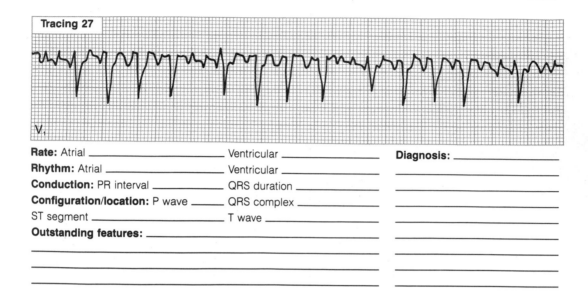

Tracing 27

V₁

Rate: Atrial _____ Ventricular _____   **Diagnosis:** _____

Rhythm: Atrial _____ Ventricular _____

Conduction: PR interval _____ QRS duration _____

Configuration/location: P wave _____ QRS complex _____

ST segment _____ T wave _____

Outstanding features: _____

_____

_____

_____

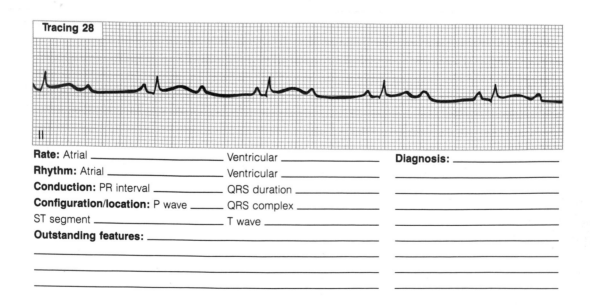

Tracing 28

II

Rate: Atrial _____ Ventricular _____   **Diagnosis:** _____

Rhythm: Atrial _____ Ventricular _____

Conduction: PR interval _____ QRS duration _____

Configuration/location: P wave _____ QRS complex _____

ST segment _____ T wave _____

Outstanding features: _____

_____

_____

_____

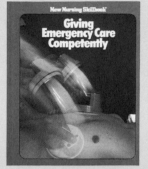
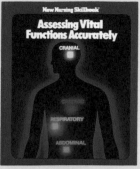
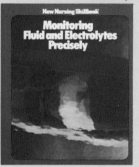
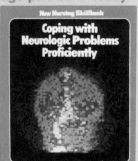
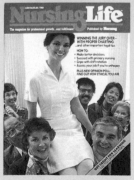

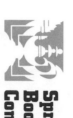

Tracing 29

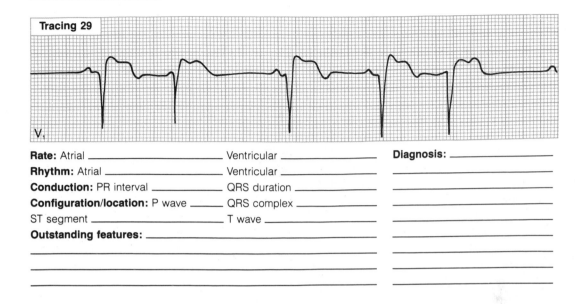

V₁

Rate: Atrial _____ Ventricular _____   **Diagnosis:** _____

Rhythm: Atrial _____ Ventricular _____   _____

Conduction: PR interval _____ QRS duration _____   _____

Configuration/location: P wave _____ QRS complex _____   _____

ST segment _____ T wave _____   _____

Outstanding features: _____   _____

_____   _____

_____   _____

_____

Tracing 30

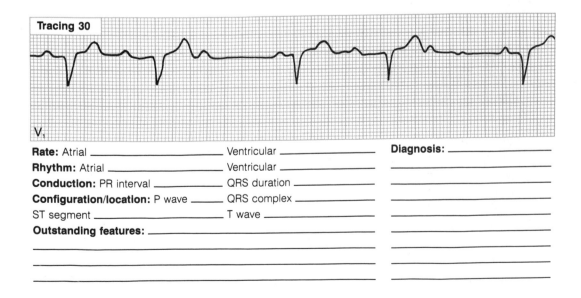

V₁

Rate: Atrial _____ Ventricular _____   **Diagnosis:** _____

Rhythm: Atrial _____ Ventricular _____   _____

Conduction: PR interval _____ QRS duration _____   _____

Configuration/location: P wave _____ QRS complex _____   _____

ST segment _____ T wave _____   _____

Outstanding features: _____   _____

_____   _____

_____   _____

_____

Tracing 31

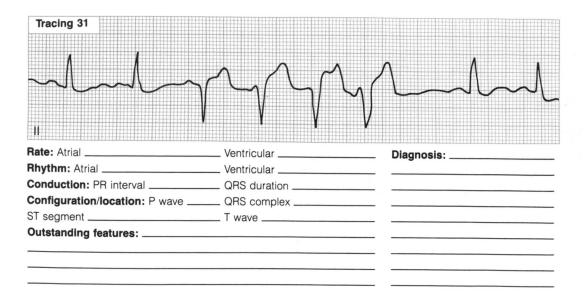

II

Rate: Atrial _____ Ventricular _____   **Diagnosis:** _____

Rhythm: Atrial _____ Ventricular _____   _____

Conduction: PR interval _____ QRS duration _____   _____

Configuration/location: P wave _____ QRS complex _____   _____

ST segment _____ T wave _____   _____

Outstanding features: _____   _____

_____   _____

_____   _____

_____   _____

Tracing 32

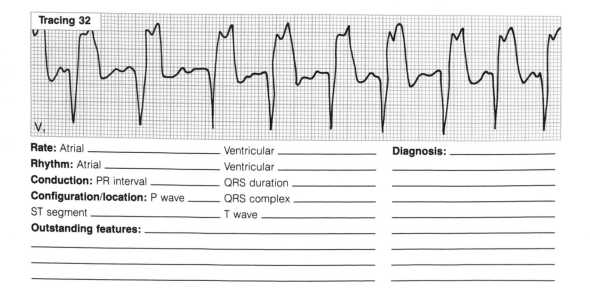

V

V₁

Rate: Atrial _____ Ventricular _____   **Diagnosis:** _____

Rhythm: Atrial _____ Ventricular _____   _____

Conduction: PR interval _____ QRS duration _____   _____

Configuration/location: P wave _____ QRS complex _____   _____

ST segment _____ T wave _____   _____

Outstanding features: _____   _____

_____   _____

_____   _____

_____   _____

Test Yourself Answers

Tracing 1

Rate: Atrial: *75;* Ventricular: *75*

Rhythm: Atrial: *regular;* Ventricular; *regular (one dropped QRS)*

Conduction: PR interval: *0.24 second;* QRS duration: *0.14 second*

Configuration/location: P wave: *configuration varies, precedes QRS;* QRS complex: *wide, prolonged;*
ST segment: *normal;* T wave: *inverted*

Outstanding features: *One dropped QRS; conduction delay through AV node and bundle branches; vary-ing configuration of P waves; inverted T waves*

Diagnosis: *Normal sinus rhythm; nonconducted PAC; first-degree heart block*

Tracing 2

Rate: Atrial: *approximately 500;* Ventricular: *approximately 100*

Rhythm: Atrial: *chaotic;* Ventricular: *irregular*

Conduction: PR interval: *not measurable;* QRS duration: *0.14 second*

Configuration/location: P wave: *merged with T waves;* QRS complex: *normal, wide;*
ST segment: *elevated;* T wave: *merged with P waves*

Outstanding features: *Rapid atrial rate; normal ventricular rate; irregular atrial and ventricular rhythms; wide QRS*

Diagnosis: *Atrial fibrillation; ventricular conduction delay*

Tracing 3

Rate: Atrial: *79;* Ventricular: *79*

Rhythm: Atrial: *regular;* Ventricular: *regular*

Conduction: PR interval: *0.20 second;* QRS duration: *0.12 second*

Configuration/location: P wave: *normal, precedes QRS;* QRS complex: *slightly widened;*
ST segment: *elevated;* T wave: *rounded*

Outstanding features: *Normal rates; normal atrial and ventricular rhythms*

Diagnosis: *Normal sinus rhythm; PVC; prolonged QRS duration*

Tracing 4

Rate: Atrial: *75;* Ventricular: *75*

Rhythm: Atrial: *slightly irregular;* Ventricular: *slightly irregular*

Conduction: PR interval: *0.16 second;* QRS duration: *0.10 second*

Configuration/location: P wave: *changes configuration, precedes QRS;* QRS complex: *normal;*
ST segment: *slightly depressed;* T wave: *rounded*

Outstanding features: *Slightly irregular atrial and ventricular rhythms; PR intervals vary slightly; P wave changes configuration*

Diagnosis: *Wandering pacemaker with junctional or low atrial premature beats*

Tracing 5

Rate: Atrial: *not measurable;* Ventricular: *not measurable*

Rhythm: Atrial: *not measurable;* Ventricular: *not measurable*

Conduction: PR interval: *not measurable;* QRS duration: *not measurable*

Configuration/location: P wave: *absent;* QRS complex: *absent;*
ST segment: *absent;* T wave: *absent*

Outstanding features: *Chaotic baseline*

Diagnosis: *Coarse ventricular fibrillation*

Tracing 6

Rate: Atrial: *65;* Ventricular: *65*

Rhythm: Atrial: *regular with PAC;* Ventricular: *regular with premature beat*

Conduction: PR interval: *0.20 second;* QRS duration: *0.10 second*

Configuration/location: P wave: *normal, precedes QRS;* QRS complex: *normal;*
ST segment: *elevated;* T wave: *peaked*

Outstanding features: *Normal atrial and ventricular rates with two premature ectopic beats (atrial); irregular ventricular rhythm (short cycles)*

Diagnosis: *Normal sinus rhythm with two premature atrial contractions*

Tracing 7

Rate: Atrial: *46;* Ventricular: *46*

Rhythm: Atrial: *regular;* Ventricular: *regular*

Conduction: PR interval: *0.16 second;* QRS duration: *0.08 second*

Configuration/location: P wave: *normal, precedes QRS;* QRS complex: *normal, follows P wave;*
ST segment: *depressed;* T wave: *slightly flat*

Outstanding features: *Slow atrial and ventricular rates*

Diagnosis: *Sinus bradycardia*

Tracing 8

Rate: Atrial: *approximately 100;* Ventricular: *approximately 100*

Rhythm: Atrial: *irregular;* Ventricular: *irregular*

Conduction: PR interval: *0.12 second;* QRS duration: *0.10 second*

Configuration/location: P wave: *normal, alternating with premature or ectopic P waves;*
QRS complex: *normal;* ST segment: *slightly elevated;* T wave: *upright*

Outstanding features: *Every QRS complex is preceded by a premature or ectopic P wave; in these cycles, apparent merging of T waves with a premature P wave*

Diagnosis: *Atrial bigeminy*

Tracing 9

Rate: Atrial: *approximately 60;* Ventricular: *approximately 60*

Rhythm: Atrial: *slightly irregular;* Ventricular: *slightly irregular*

Conduction: PR interval: *0.24 second;* QRS duration: *0.10 second*

Configuration/location: P wave: *normal, precedes QRS;* QRS complex: *normal, follows P wave;* ST segment: *elevated;* T wave: *rounded*

Outstanding features: *Slow atrial and ventricular rate; slightly irregular atrial and ventricular rhythms; prolonged PR interval (AV conduction delay)*

Diagnosis: *Sinus bradycardia; sinus arrhythmia; first-degree heart block*

Tracing 10

Rate: Atrial: *60;* Ventricular: *60*

Rhythm: Atrial: *regular;* Ventricular: *slightly irregular*

Conduction: PR interval: *0.20 second;* QRS duration: *0.10 second*

Configuration/location: P wave: *flat, precedes QRS;* QRS complex: *normal;* ST segment: *depressed;* T wave: *upright*

Outstanding features: *Slow atrial and ventricular rates; regular atrial rhythm and irregular ventricular rhythm; one wide, premature, bizarre QRS*

Diagnosis: *Sinus bradycardia; PVC interpolated*

Tracing 11

Rate: Atrial: *83;* Ventricular: *83*

Rhythm: Atrial: *regular;* Ventricular: *regular*

Conduction: PR interval: *0.16 second;* QRS duration: *0.22 second*

Configuration/location: P wave: *peaked, precedes most QRS;* QRS complex: *wide;* ST segment: *elevated;* T wave: *normal*

Outstanding features: *Normal atrial and ventricular rates; regular atrial and ventricular rhythms; wide QRS complexes, one of which is distorted*

Diagnosis: *Normal sinus rhythm with PVC and right bundle branch block*

Tracing 12

Rate: Atrial: *approximately 500;* Ventricular: *approximately 88*

Rhythm: Atrial: *irregular;* Ventricular: *irregular*

Conduction: PR interval: *not measurable;* QRS duration: *0.08 second*

Configuration/location: P wave (fibrillation waves): *merged with T wave;* QRS complex: *normal;* ST segment: *not measurable;* T wave: *merged with P wave*

Outstanding features: *Rapid atrial rate; irregular ventricular rhythm; no measurable PR interval*

Diagnosis: *Atrial fibrillation*

Tracing 13
Rate: Atrial: *not measurable;* Ventricular: *250*
Rhythm: Atrial: *not measurable;* Ventricular: *regular*
Conduction: PR interval: *not measurable;* QRS duration: *0.24 second*
Configuration/location: P wave: *absent;* QRS complex: *wide, bizarre;*
ST segment: *none;* T wave: *absent*
Outstanding features: *Chaotic baseline; no discernible complexes*
Diagnosis: *Ventricular tachycardia*

Tracing 14
Rate: Atrial: *not present;* Ventricular: *72*
Rhythm: Atrial: *not measurable;* Ventricular: *regular*
Conduction: PR interval: *not measurable;* QRS duration: *0.08 second*
Configuration/location: P wave: *absent;* QRS complex: *normal;*
ST segment: *depressed;* T wave: *upright*
Outstanding features: *Absent P waves; regular ventricular rhythm*
Diagnosis: *Junctional tachycardia*

Tracing 15
Rate: Atrial: *43 (sinus beats);* Ventricular: *43 (sinus beats)*
Rhythm: Atrial: *not measurable;* Ventricular: *irregular*
Conduction: PR interval: *0.18 second;* QRS duration: *0.12 second*
Configuration/location: P wave: *rounded, precedes some QRS;* QRS complex: *distorted;*
ST segment: *depressed;* T wave: *inverted*
Outstanding features: *Every other QRS complex wide, bizarre, and premature*
Diagnosis: *Ventricular bigeminy with normal sinus rhythm*

Tracing 16
Rate: Atrial: *not measurable;* Ventricular: *not measurable*
Rhythm: Atrial: *not measurable;* Ventricular: *not measurable*
Conduction: PR interval: *not measurable;* QRS duration: *not measurable*
Configuration/location: P wave: *absent;* QRS complex: *absent;*
ST segment: *absent;* T wave: *absent*
Outstanding features: *Undulating, chaotic baseline; no distinguishing features*
Diagnosis: *Ventricular fibrillation*

Tracing 17

Rate: Atrial: *375;* Ventricular: *approximately 75*

Rhythm: Atrial: *irregular;* Ventricular: *irregular*

Conduction: PR interval: *not measurable;* QRS duration: *0.08 second*

Configuration/location: P wave: *lost in T wave;* QRS complex: *normal;*
ST segment: *not measurable;* T wave: *merged with P wave*

Outstanding features: *Rapid atrial rate; ventricular rate slower than atrial rate; no measurable PR interval; irregular atrial and ventricular rhythms; P waves and T waves merged to form uneven baseline*

Diagnosis: *Atrial flutter — fibrillation or course atrial fibrillation*

Tracing 18

Rate: Atrial: *88;* Ventricular: *88*

Rhythm: Atrial: *regular;* Ventricular: *regular with one short cycle*

Conduction: PR interval: *0.16 second;* QRS duration: *0.08 second*

Configuration/location: P wave: *normal, precedes QRS;* QRS complex: *normal, follows P wave;*
ST segment: *slightly elevated;* T wave: *inverted*

Outstanding features: *Normal atrial and ventricular rates; regular atrial rhythm; regular ventricular rhythm with one short cycle*

Diagnosis: *Normal sinus rhythm with premature atrial contraction*

Tracing 19

Rate: Atrial: *83;* Ventricular: *83*

Rhythm: Atrial: *irregular;* Ventricular: *irregular*

Conduction: PR interval: *0.16 second;* QRS duration: *0.12 second*

Configuration/location: P wave: *normal, precedes QRS;* QRS complex: *normal, follows P wave;*
ST segment: *elevated;* T wave: *rounded*

Outstanding features: *Slightly irregular atrial and ventricular rhythms; long pause with dropped QRS complex that was not preceded by a P wave; one short RR interval with PR interval less than patient's normal PR interval*

Diagnosis: *Normal sinus rhythm; premature atrial contraction; sinus arrest*

Tracing 20

Rate: Atrial: *not measurable;* Ventricular: *not measurable*

Rhythm: Atrial: *not measurable;* Ventricular: *not measurable*

Conduction: PR interval: *not measurable;* QRS duration: *not measurable*

Configuration/location: P wave: *not visible;* QRS complex: *not measurable;*
ST segment: *not measurable;* T wave: *not measurable*

Outstanding features: *Chaotic rhythm with no discernible characteristics*

Diagnosis: *Ventricular fibrillation*

Tracing 21

Rate: Atrial: *approximately 500;* Ventricular: *approximately 115*

Rhythm: Atrial: *irregular;* Ventricular: *irregular*

Conduction: PR interval: *not measurable;* QRS duration: *0.10 second*

Configuration/location: P wave: *merged with T waves;* QRS complex: *normal;*
ST segment: *normal;* T wave: *merged with P waves*

Outstanding features: *Rapid, irregular atrial rate; slightly rapid ventricular rate; irregular atrial and ventricular rhythms*

Diagnosis: *Atrial fibrillation*

Tracing 22

Rate: Atrial: *approximately 500;* Ventricular: *approximately 88*

Rhythm: Atrial: *irregular;* Ventricular: *irregular*

Conduction: PR interval: *not measurable;* QRS duration: *0.10 second*

Configuration/location: P wave: *merged with T wave;* QRS complex: *normal;*
ST segment: *slightly depressed;* T wave: *merged with P wave*

Outstanding features: *Rapid atrial rate; irregular atrial and ventricular rhythms*

Diagnosis: *Atrial fibrillation*

Tracing 23

Rate: Atrial: *79;* Ventricular: *79*

Rhythm: Atrial: *regular;* Ventricular: *regular*

Conduction: PR interval: *0.24 second;* QRS duration: *0.16 second*

Configuration/location: P wave: *normal, precedes QRS;* QRS complex: *wide, follows P wave;*
ST segment: *normal;* T wave: *inverted*

Outstanding features: *Normal atrial and ventricular rates; regular atrial and ventricular rhythms; prolonged PR interval and QRS duration*

Diagnosis: *Normal sinus rhythm; first-degree block; PVC; right bundle branch block*

Tracing 24

Rate: Atrial: *107;* Ventricular: *107*

Rhythm: Atrial: *not measurable;* Ventricular: *regular*

Conduction: PR interval: *not measurable;* QRS duration: *0.11 second*

Configuration/location: P wave: *absent;* QRS complex: *normal;*
ST segment: *slightly depressed;* T wave: *inverted*

Outstanding features: *Absent P waves; regular ventricular rhythm*

Diagnosis: *Junctional tachycardia*

Tracing 25

Rate: Atrial: *94;* Ventricular: *94*

Rhythm: Atrial: *fairly regular;* Ventricular: *irregular*

Conduction: PR interval: *0.20 second;* QRS duration: *0.08 second*

Configuration/location: P wave: *low, rounded, precedes most QRS complexes;* QRS complex: *normal, two of which are wide and distorted;* ST segment: *elevated;* T wave: *rounded*

Outstanding features: *Normal atrial and ventricular rates; irregular ventricular rhythm; two distorted and wide QRS complexes*

Diagnosis: *Normal sinus rhythm with PVCs*

Tracing 26

Rate: Atrial: *88;* Ventricular: *88*

Rhythm: Atrial: *regular;* Ventricular: *regular*

Conduction: PR interval: *0.18 second;* QRS duration: *0.14 second*

Configuration/location: P wave: *low, precedes QRS;* QRS complex: *wide, follows P wave;* ST segment: *depressed;* T wave: *flat*

Outstanding features: *Prolonged QRS duration*

Diagnosis: *Normal sinus rhythm; left bundle branch block*

Tracing 27

Rate: Atrial: *300;* Ventricular: *136*

Rhythm: Atrial: *regular;* Ventricular: *irregular*

Conduction: PR interval: *not measurable;* QRS duration: *0.08 second*

Configuration/location: P wave ("flutter" wave): *merged with T wave;* QRS complex: *normal;* ST segment: *elevated;* T wave: *merged with P wave*

Outstanding features: *Rapid atrial and ventricular rates; irregular ventricular rhythm*

Diagnosis: *Atrial flutter — 2:1 and 4:1; AV conduction*

Tracing 28

Rate: Atrial: *94;* Ventricular: *47*

Rhythm: Atrial: *regular;* Ventricular: *regular*

Conduction: PR interval: *0.20 second;* QRS duration: *0.10 second*

Configuration/location: P wave: *normal, precedes QRS;* QRS complex: *normal, some absent;* ST segment: *elevated;* T wave: *upright*

Outstanding features: *Atrial rate twice the ventricular rate; two P waves for every QRS complex; consistent PR interval*

Diagnosis: *Second-degree AV block — 2:1*

Tracing 29

Rate: Atrial: *58;* Ventricular: *approximately 58*

Rhythm: Atrial: *irregular;* Ventricular: *irregular*

Conduction: PR interval: *0.16 second;* QRS duration: *0.12 second*

Configuration/location: P wave: normal, absent in shorter cycles; QRS complex: *normal;*
ST segment: *elevated;* T wave: *normal*

Outstanding features: *Irregular ventricular rhythm caused by short cycles; P waves absent in short cycles*

Diagnosis: *Normal sinus rhythm with premature junctional beats*

Tracing 30

Rate: Atrial: *72;* Ventricular: *39 to 63 (depends on block)*

Rhythm: Atrial: *slightly irregular;* Ventricular: *irregular*

Conduction: PR interval: *varies;* QRS duration: *0.08 to 0.09 second*

Configuration/location: P wave: *rounded, precedes QRS;* QRS complex: *broad, some absent;*
ST segment: *elevated;* T wave: *rounded*

Outstanding features: *Three P waves for every two QRS complexes; PR varies; ventricular rate and rhythm vary with degree of block*

Diagnosis: *Second-degree block — (Wenckebach 3:2 conduction)*

Tracing 31

Rate: Atrial: *83;* Ventricular: *83*

Rhythm: Atrial: *regular;* Ventricular: *fairly regular*

Conduction: PR interval: *0.18 second;* QRS duration: *0.12 second*

Configuration/location: P wave: *some flat, some varying shapes, some absent, usually precede QRS;* QRS complex: *slightly wide, changes direction in some beats;*
ST segment: *depressed and elevated;* T wave: *rounded and peaked*

Outstanding features: *Normal heart rates; regular atrial rhythm; slightly irregular ventricular rhythm; prolonged QRS duration*

Diagnosis: *Normal sinus rhythm; short run of slow ventricular tachycardia*

Tracing 32

Rate: Atrial: *approximately 500;* Ventricular: *approximately 100*

Rhythm: Atrial: *chaotic, irregular;* Ventricular: *irregular*

Conduction: PR interval: *not measurable;* QRS duration: *0.10 second*

Configuration/location: P wave: *merged with T waves;* QRS complex: *normal;*
ST segment: *elevated;* T wave: *merged with P waves*

Outstanding features: *Different atrial and ventricular rates; irregular atrial rhythm (chaotic baseline); irregular ventricular rhythm; merged P waves and T waves to form fibrillation waves*

Diagnosis: *Atrial fibrillation*

SKILLCHECK ANSWERS

ANSWERS TO SKILLCHECK 1 (page 31)

1. Atrial and ventricular rates are 60; both rhythms are regular. The PR interval measures 0.18 second, and the QRS duration measures 0.10 second. P waves are inverted but precede the QRS complexes. QRS complexes are normal. ST segments are depressed, and T waves are biphasic.

2. Atrial and ventricular rates are 52; both rhythms are regular. The PR interval measures 0.20 second, and the QRS duration measures 0.12 second. P waves are flat but always precede the QRS complexes. QRS complexes are normal, as are the ST segments. T waves are upright.

ANSWERS TO SKILLCHECK 2 (pages 77-81)

1. Normal sinus rhythm. This tracing is normal in rate (90), rhythm (regular), conduction (0.17 second for the PR interval, 0.08 second for the QRS duration), and configuration of the QRS complex. (P waves and T waves are slightly rounded, and the ST segments slightly depressed; see Chapter 9 for an explanation.)

2. Sinus tachycardia. Rates in this tracing are rapid (120). However, the rhythm is regular, the PR interval is normal (0.18 second), and the QRS duration is normal (0.08 second). (Notice the slight abnormalities in wave configuration — rounded P waves, coved T waves, and an elevated ST segment. See Chapter 9 for an explanation.)

3. Sinus bradycardia with premature atrial contraction. The atrial and ventricular rhythms are slightly irregular, with one short cycle.

4. Atrial fibrillation. The atrial rate is difficult to measure in this tracing. Atrial rhythm is irregular, and ventricular rhythm is grossly irregular. P waves and T waves form an uneven baseline.

5. Atrial flutter. Atrial rate is 300. Ventricular rhythm is irregular. P waves and T waves have merged to form sawtooth "F" (flutter) waves.

6. Junctional tachycardia. P waves are absent. QRS complex is normal. Ventricular rate is 70.

7. Junctional rhythm. P waves are absent, but the QRS is normal. The ventricular rate is 40.

8. Normal sinus rhythm with first-degree block. The PR interval is prolonged (0.28 second).

9. Second-degree block (Wenckebach). The PR interval varies. Ventricular rate varies from 35 to 56, and ventricular rhythm varies with the block (2:1/3:2 conduction).

10. Second-degree block, Mobitz II (2:1). The PR interval is consistent, but the QRS complex is dropped after every other P wave.

11. Normal sinus rhythm with premature ventricular contraction. Two QRS complexes deflect in the opposite direction from normal. T waves following the abnormal QRS complexes also deflect in the opposite direction. A compensatory pause follows the abnormal complexes.

12. Asystole. The baseline shows only minimal activity (small waves of excitability appear to come from chest compression).

13. Normal sinus rhythm with premature ventricular contraction. One QRS complex is wide and distorted. The P wave preceding it is flat but not premature. There is a compensatory pause after the distorted QRS.

14. Ventricular tachycardia. The QRS complexes are wide and bizarre and occur in rapid succession.

ANSWERS TO SKILLCHECK 3 (pages 107-111)

1a to 1c. Infarction of the inferior wall. Leads II, III, and aVF face the inferior surface of the heart. The presence of Q waves and flattened T waves indicates an infarction of the inferior wall of the heart.

2a to 2c. Muscle injury and ischemia of the anterior wall. Leads I, V_2, and V_3 face the anterior surface of the heart. Slight depression on the ST segments and inversion of the T waves indicate injury to the anterior myocardium, with resultant ischemia.

3a to 3c. Current of injury of the inferior wall. Leads II, III, and aVF face the inferior surface of the heart. Elevation of the ST segments indicates a current of injury, which indicates possible ischemia of the inferior wall of the heart.

4. Muscle tremors.

5. Electrical interference (60-cycle alternating current) and muscle movement.

6. Muscle movement.

7. Electrical interference (60-cycle alternating current).

8. Wandering baseline due to respiratory movement.

Appendices

CALCULATING HEART RATE

If you're calculating your patient's atrial rate, count the blocks between consecutive P waves; for ventricular rate, count between consecutive R waves. Then, check this chart to determine heart rate. *Note:* This chart is based on a standard of 1,500 small EKG squares/minute. Use this calculation method for *regular rhythm only.* Paper speed is 25 mm/second.

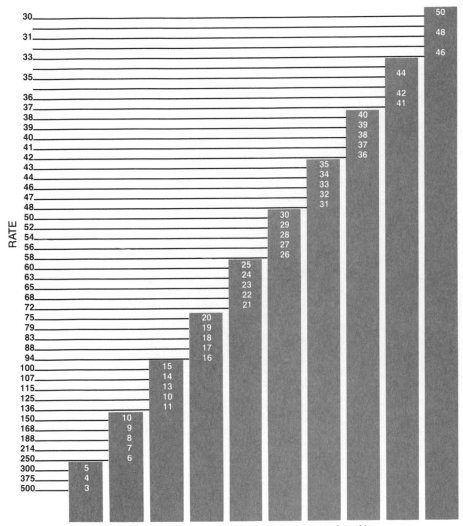

NUMBER OF SMALL SQUARES (0.04 second each)

ATRIAL DYSRHYTHMIAS

RHYTHM	MECHANISM AND FEATURES
Normal sinus rhythm	SA node acts as pacemaker. Impulses travel through the normal conduction paths. *EKG features:* Heart rate is 60 to 100 beats/minute (regular rhythm). P wave precedes each QRS complex. PR interval is normal.
Sinus bradycardia	Same as normal sinus rhythm except heart rate is below 60 beats/minute.
Sinus tachycardia	Same as normal sinus rhythm except heart rate is over 100 beats/minute but less than 160.
Sinus arrhythmia	SA node acts as pacemaker, but heart rate changes periodically. Heart rate increases with inspiration or decreases with expiration (common in children). *EKG features:* RR intervals are irregular; PP intervals vary slightly.
Wandering atrial pacemaker	SA node remains as basic pacemaker, but heart may also be paced by random atrial foci or AV node. *EKG features:* Ventricular rhythm varies. P waves change configuration or are absent for some beats; PR interval varies.
Sinus arrest (atrial standstill, sinus pause)	Momentary failure of the SA node to initiate an impulse. May be caused by pharyngeal irritation, increased vagal stimulation, anesthesia intubation, carotid sinus massage, or deep inspiration. Cause may be unknown. *EKG features:* Normal sinus rhythm interrupted by an occasional long pause where an entire cardiac cycle (P, QRS, T) is missing. RR intervals vary because pause isn't equal to two regular cycles.
SA block	Impulse from SA node fails to reach atria; no atrial or ventricular contractions. *EKG features:* Normal sinus rhythm interrupted by an occasional long pause where entire cardiac cycle (P, QRS, T) is missing. Rhythm remains normal because pause is equal to two regular cycles.

	SIGNIFICANCE	TREATMENT
	Conduction system is operating normally.	None.
	May be normal in athletes but could also indicate atrial disease or myocardial anoxia. Cardiac output is reduced.	If symptomatic, treat with atropine, isoproterenol, or pacemaker.
	Nonspecific; depends on cause (fever, emotional upset, or activity).	Usually none.
	Innocent disturbance of the normal pacemaker or caused by hyperventilation.	Usually none. Observe patient for other atrial dysrhythmias.
	Can occur in normal heart from increased vagal tone. Often found in rheumatic carditis due to tissue inflammation.	Usually none. Determine cause and treat if necessary.
	Important if caused by vagal reactions, such as fainting, dizziness, or syncope. Can be caused by digitalis or quinidine excess.	Determine and treat cause. In cases where the patient is symptomatic with syncope, assist with the insertion of a pacemaker.
	May indicate excess of digitalis or quinidine, vagal stimulation (for example, carotid massage), or organic heart disease near SA node.	Usually none. Determine cause.

(Continued on next page)

ATRIAL DYSRHYTHMIAS (continued)

RHYTHM	MECHANISM AND FEATURES
Premature atrial contractions (PACs)	An irritable focus in the atria supercedes the SA node as pacemaker for one or more beats. Ventricular conduction is normal. *EKG features:* P waves differ in shape; may be inverted, notched, slurred, flat, or diphasic. P waves also change location, merging with T waves or with QRS complexes.
Paroxysmal atrial tachycardia (PAT)	An irritable focus in the atria increases rate to 160 to 250 beats/minute. Onset of PAT is always sudden. *EKG features:* P waves may be hidden in QRS, eliminating PR interval. Rhythm is perfectly regular.
Atrial flutter	An irritable focus in the atria takes over pacing. *EKG features:* Atrial rate is 250 to 350 beats/minute; ventricular rate varies with degree of block in AV conduction. P waves become superimposed on T waves as atrial rate increases, causing a wavy or sawtooth configuration between QRS complexes.
Atrial fibrillation	An atrial ectopic focus discharges more than 400 impulses/minute. Atria lose ability to contract uniformly; atrial walls twitch rather than contract. Only a small percentage of atrial stimuli reaches ventricles. *EKG features:* Ventricular rhythm is irregular. P waves and T waves are replaced by small, irregular, chaotic waves ("f" or fibrillatory waves). QRS complexes are normal in shape and duration (if bundle branch block isn't present) but occur irregularly (RR intervals vary.)

DYSRHYTHMIAS OF THE AV NODE

RHYTHM	MECHANISM AND FEATURES
Premature junctional contractions; premature nodal contractions (PNCs)	The AV node replaces the SA node as the pacemaker; impulses originate in AV node. Impulse is transmitted to the ventricles and then upward to the atria (retrograde conduction). *EKG features:* P waves may not be visible, or they occur before or after QRS complexes, depending on relative speeds of retrograde conduction; PR intervals are less than 0.10 second.
Junctional rhythm	Impulses arise in the AV node and control both the ventricles and atria because they spread in both directions. *EKG features:* P waves have the characteristics of PNCs. QRS duration is usually normal. Ventricular rates range from 40 to 60 beats/minute.

	SIGNIFICANCE	TREATMENT
	Dangerous only if more than 6 to 10 beats/minute; may develop into paroxysmal atrial tachycardia or atrial fibrillation. Often caused by excess alcohol, tobacco, or food.	If cause is organic, treat disease. Give potassium supplement, as well as digitalis or quinidine.
	Serious in organic heart disease. Can cause congestive heart failure or angina if underlying heart disease is present.	Give verapamil I.V. Carotid massage may be applied by the doctor.
	Atria aren't contracting normally. May cause congestive heart failure.	Give digitalis to convert flutter to fibrillation or normal sinus rhythm; then quinidine to treat fibrillation or maintain normal sinus rhythm. Other treatments include propranolol or direct-current shock (cardioversion).
	Seen in hyperthyroidism or organic heart disease. Reduces cardiac efficiency by reducing cardiac output. May cause atrial thrombi, increasing risk of embolism.	Give digitalis, quinidine, or propranolol. Other treatment includes direct-current shock (cardioversion). (Atrial fibrillation is under control when ventricular rate is under 100.)

	SIGNIFICANCE	TREATMENT
	Same as PACs.	Usually none. May give potassium or propranolol. Watch for junctional tachycardia.
	Can result from excess of digitalis or quinidine. In organic heart disease, rhythm may be permanent.	Correct serum potassium levels.

(Continued on next page)

DYSRHYTHMIAS OF THE AV NODE *(continued)*

RHYTHM	MECHANISM AND FEATURES
Junctional tachycardia	Ventricular rate is 60 to 200 beats/minute and may be paroxysmal. *EKG features:* Tracing resembles junctional rhythm except the ventricular rate ranges from 60 to 100 (slow junctional tachycardia) to 100 to 220 (rapid junctional tachycardia).

HEART BLOCK

RHYTHM	MECHANISM AND FEATURES
First-degree (1°) AV block	Conduction is normal to the AV node, but delayed through the AV node. *EKG features:* PR intervals are prolonged to more than 0.21 second.
Second-degree (2°) AV block	*Wenckebach (Mobitz I):* *EKG features:* PR intervals vary, becoming progressively longer until a QRS is dropped. Usually there is a cyclic pattern to dropped beats (4:1, 5:1). *Mobitz II* *EKG features:* PR intervals are fixed, but periodically QRS is dropped. *2:1* *EKG features:* Every other QRS is dropped.
Third-degree (3°) AV block	Impulses from the atria to the ventricles are blocked, so the atria and ventricles beat independently of each other. There are two pacemakers — one in the atria and one in the ventricles. *EKG features:* Atrial rate is higher than the ventricular rate (ventricular rate is 20 to 40 beats/minute) and is usually regular. P waves are unrelated to QRS complexes. PR intervals vary.
AV dissociation	Mechanism is the same as third-degree block except there is no heart block. There are two pacemakers — one in the atria and the other in the AV node. *EKG features:* Ventricular rate is higher than the atrial rate because ventricles are stimulated from AV node or ventricles. P waves are unrelated to QRS complexes. PR intervals vary or are absent.

	SIGNIFICANCE	TREATMENT
	Ventricular rates over 150 beats/minute usually caused by excess of digitalis. Can cause congestive heart failure.	Give potassium, propranolol, small doses of digitalis. Also direct-current shock (cardioversion) if patient's hemodynamically collapsed.

	SIGNIFICANCE	TREATMENT
	Least dangerous of AV blocks. May be produced by drugs (digitalis and quinidine).	Observe patient for advancing block.
 Mobitz II	In 2° block, a narrow QRS means a block in the AV node; a wide QRS means a block below the bundle of His. Dropped beats mean the ventricles aren't contracting rhythmically. Cardiac output may be impaired. Ventricular rate is affected by degree of block. 2:1 block may be highly dangerous because of a slow ventricular rate.	Treatment depends on the cause and width of QRS complexes; may require permanent pacing if QRS is wide. Other treatment includes atropine or isoproterenol or stopping digitalis.
	Causes poor perfusion, Stokes-Adams attacks, PVCs, or ventricular fibrillation.	Doctor must insert a permanent pacemaker.
	Can be caused by digitalis toxicity or disease. Determine cause.	If cause is from digitalis toxicity, discontinue digitalis. May give atropine to increase the atrial rate by speeding the sinus node or assist in inserting a temporary pacemaker. However, usually no treatment is required.

VENTRICULAR DYSRHYTHMIAS

RHYTHM	MECHANISM AND FEATURES
Bundle branch block (BBB)	Conduction is normal from SA node through the AV node where it is obstructed in one of the branches. Conduction through the right or left branches of the bundle of His is impaired. *EKG features:* QRS is widened to 0.12 second or greater.
Premature ventricular contraction (PVC)	Ectopic focus in ventricles stimulates heart before the regularly scheduled SA impulse arrives. *EKG features:* P wave may or may not be seen. QRS is wide, premature, bizarre, often going in a different direction from patient's normal QRS. T wave is in opposite direction from QRS.
Ventricular tachycardia	Ventricles are repeatedly stimulated by ectopic foci. This dysrhythmia may develop spontaneously but usually occurs with PVCs. *EKG features:* When there are 3 PVCs in a row, ventricular tachycardia exists. P waves may or may not be seen. QRS is wide and bizarre. Rhythm is usually regular, but there may be a slight irregularity.
Ventricular flutter	This dysrhythmia appears minutes or seconds before ventricular fibrillation or may follow ventricular tachycardia. *EKG features:* Many multifocal, bizarre PVCs appear. Tracing becomes a wavy, sawtooth configuration with no discernible P, QRS, or T waves.
Ventricular fibrillation	Ventricles are repeatedly stimulated from an ectopic focus so rapidly that the heart can't recover after contractions. *EKG features:* Tracing becomes a series of chaotic waves with no uniformity.
Cardiac arrest (ventricular standstill or asystole)	There is no cardiac electrical activity. Ventricles cease to contract. *EKG features:* Tracing becomes a flat line.

	SIGNIFICANCE	TREATMENT
	May occur in normal patients and cause no symptoms, but left BBB is more likely associated with underlying heart disease.	Usually none. If complicated by advanced AVB, though, assist with the insertion of a pacemaker.
	Reflects ventricular irritability. Frequency of occurrence indicates degree of irritability. Dangerous when PVCs are multifocal (coming from more than one focus), or in clusters (2 or more), or when showing R on T pattern.	Give lidocaine bolus and drip, procainamide, quinidine, or phenytoin.
	Often precedes ventricular fibrillation. May be transient and self-terminating. If sustained may lead to ventricular fibrillation, congestive failure, and cardiogenic shock. May be mistaken for atrial fibrillation or supraventricular tachycardia with aberrency (wide QRS) or WPW.	Treatment depends on patient's reaction. If run of ventricular tachycardia is short, give drugs as for PVCs or assist with the insertion of a temporary pacemaker for overdrive suppression. If run is sustained, direct-current shock (cardioversion) may have to be administered.
	Lethal dysrhythmia	Administer direct-current shock (cardioversion).
	Most serious of all dysrhythmias. Must treat PVCs and ventricular tachycardia to prevent ventricular fibrillation. Must be differentiated from ventricular tachycardia or standstill.	Repeatedly apply direct-current shock (cardioversion) until dysrhythmia is reversed. Follow with lidocaine and, if necessary, CPR.
	May be caused by acute MI; terminal illness; excess digitalis, quinidine, procainamide, or lidocaine; or by straining at defecation.	Give a sharp blow to the chest and administer CPR. Give intracardiac epinephrine. Assist with insertion of a transvenous pacemaker.

ANTIARRHYTHMIC AGENTS

GENERIC NAME	TRADE NAME	DOSE
quinidine	Cardioquin Quinaglute Quinidex Quinora	200 to 300 mg q 4 to 6 hours, P.O. (Some preparations are q 8 hours or q 12 hours.)
procainamide	Procan SR Pronestyl Pronestyl SR	250 to 1,000 mg q 3 to 6 hours, P.O.; 0.5 to 1 g q 4 to 6 hours, I.M.; 2 to 6 mg/minute I.V. infusion
lidocaine	Xylocaine	50 to 100 mg I.V. bolus; repeat in 5 to 10 minutes; then 1 to 4 mg/minute I.V. infusion
phenytoin	Dilantin	250 to 500 mg slow I.V. push, then 200 to 300 mg q.i.d. or b.i.d.
propranolol	Inderal	1 to 3 mg I.V. (higher doses have been used); 10 to 40 mg q.i.d., P.O.)
verapamil	Calan Isoptin	5 to 10 mg I.V. push over 60 seconds with EKG and blood pressure monitoring. Repeat dose in 30 minutes if no response. Follow bolus injection with maintenance infusion of 0.005 mg/kg/minute.

DIGITALIS GLYCOSIDES

GENERIC NAME	TRADE NAME	DIGITALIZATION DOSE	MAINTENANCE DOSE
digitoxin	Crystodigin Purodigin	1.2 to 2 mg P.O.; 1 to 2 mg I.V or I.M.	0.05 to 0.2 mg P.O.
digoxin	Lanoxicaps Lanoxin	0.75 to 1.25 mg P.O.; 0.6 to 1 mg I.V. or I.M.	0.125 to 0.5 mg P.O.
deslanoside	Cedilanid-D	1.2 to 1.6 mg I.V. or I.M.	No oral dose

ADVERSE EFFECTS	EKG CHANGES
Cinchonism (nausea and vomiting, diarrhea, tinnitus, salivation, vertigo, visual disturbances), thrombocytopenia, rash, hypotension, fever	*Normal:* widened QRS complexes (up to 25% of normal). *Abnormal:* 2° or complete block, PVCs, ventricular dysrhythmias, QRS widening greater than 25% of normal
GI and CNS disturbances, hypotension, bone marrow depression, agranulocytosis, fever, allergic reactions, systemic lupus erythematosus–like syndrome (positive LE prep)	*Normal:* widened QRS complex *Abnormal:* tachycardia, QRS widening greater than 25% of normal
Drowsiness, CNS disturbances, convulsions (give diazepam, 10 mg I.V.), hypotension	*Abnormal:* heart block
Hypotension, CNS disturbances, rash, hyperplasia of gums	*Abnormal:* heart block, bradycardia
Heart failure, hypotension, bronchoconstriction, GI and CNS disturbances, rash, paresthesias, hypoglycemia, bradycardia	*Normal:* none *Abnormal:* heart block, bradycardia
Hypotension, CHF, bradycardia, dizziness, constipation	*Abnormal:* 3° heart block

ADVERSE EFFECTS	EKG CHANGES
Mental depression, anorexia, nausea, vomiting, restlessness, yellow vision, mental confusion, disorientation, delirium	*Normal:* prolonged PR interval *Abnormal:* PACs, PVCs, ventricular and supraventricular tachycardias, heart block, AV dissociation, junctional rhythm
Same as digitoxin	Same as digitoxin
Same as digitoxin	Same as digitoxin

Glossary

anoxia: A deficiency of oxygen in body tissues, due to reduction in blood flow or other causes.

arrhythmia: Irregularity or absence of heartbeat. See *dysrhythmia*.

asystole (cardiac arrest, ventricular standstill): The absence of a heartbeat.

atherosclerosis: The most common form of arteriosclerosis in which deposits of yellow, fatty plaques build up in the arteries; may cause arterial occlusion.

atrioventricular block: A cardiac impulse conduction disturbance in the atrioventricular node, bundle of His, or its branches.

bigeminy: Any condition that occurs in pairs, particularly two beats of the pulse in rapid succession followed by a pause.

bradycardia: A slow heart rate.

bundle branch block: An abnormality in cardiac impulse conduction through the fibers of the bundle of His.

cardiac output: Amount of blood discharged by either ventricle per minute.

cardioversion: Conversion of a dysrhythmia to normal sinus rhythm by electrical shocks or drug therapy.

carotid sinus: A dilated portion of the common carotid artery, just above the bifurcation of the two main branches containing a rich supply of nerve endings from the sinus branch of the vagus nerve.

carotid sinus pressure (or massage): Manual pressure applied on the carotid sinus; this slows the heart rate.

circus movement: The theory that an electrical impulse originates in one area, travels in a circular path, and reenters in the same area to produce a cycle (a possible mechanism for atrial flutter and fibrillation).

compensatory pause: The period following a PVC during which the heart regulates itself, allowing the SA node to resume normal conduction.

conduction time: The interval between the origination of an impulse at the SA node and the stimulation of ventricular contraction.

congestive heart failure: Failure of the heart to maintain adequate blood circulation, causing breathlessness, weakness, and abnormal sodium and water retention. This condition is caused by heart disease and may cause congestion in the lungs or in peripheral circulation.

coronary visualization (cardiac angiography): X-ray examination of the coronary arteries after a radiopaque dye has been injected into them.

dysrhythmia: Any disturbance in the normal rhythm of the heartbeat; irregularities may occur in discharge of impulses from the SA node or in conduction of impulses through heart tissue.

ectopic focus: A focus other than the normal one. In cardiology, a source of cardiac stimulus other than the SA node, usually caused by some irritation of the myocardium.

EKG (or ECG): Electrocardiogram; a graphic tracing of electrical activity of the heart.

extrasystole: A contraction of the heart that occurs prematurely and interrupts the normal rhythm.

fibrillation: Quivering or uncoordinated muscle contraction.

heart block: Impairment of cardiac conduction so that electrical impulses from the atria fail to pass through the AV node to the ventricles.

hypoxia: Low oxygen content.

infarct: Localized tissue death caused by prolonged ischemia to the area. Myocardial infarction refers to an infarct of the heart muscle.

ischemia: Localized deficiency of blood caused by constriction or obstruction of the blood vessel to the area.

junctional dysrhythmia: The irregular heartbeat that results when the AV node assumes the SA node's role as the heart's primary pacemaker.

MI: Myocardial infarction; infarct of the myocardium, usually resulting from occlusion of a coronary artery.

mitral stenosis: Stricture or narrowing of the mitral valve or orifice; usually caused by rheumatic heart disease.

Mobitz Type I (Wenckebach) block: Second-degree or partial AV block in which the PR interval increases progressively until there is no atrial impulse and the corresponding ventricular beat drops out.

Mobitz Type II block: Second-degree or partial AV block characterized by the sudden nonconduction of an atrial impulse and a periodic dropped beat that occurs without warning — without previous lengthening of the PR interval.

pacemaker: The SA node, so called because it initiates the electrical impulses that set the rhythm of cardiac contractions. An *artificial pacemaker* is an electrical device to pace cardiac rhythm, used particularly when a patient has symptomatic heart block.

parasystole: A dysrhythmia caused by two foci, usually the SA node and an ectopic focus in the ventricle, independently initiating cardiac impulses.

paroxysmal: Recurring suddenly and abruptly.

rule of bigeminy: The theory that PVCs tend to occur with low heart rates.

sinus arrhythmia: A slight variation or irregularity in sinus rhythm, or normal heartbeats.

Stokes-Adams syndrome: Sudden attacks of unconsciousness, sometimes coupled with convulsions, which may accompany heart block or ventricular dysrhythmia both producing low cardiac outputs.

systole: Contraction of the heart, which causes ejection of blood from the heart chambers into the circulatory system.

tachycardia: A fast heart rate.

vagal stimulation: Pharmacologic or manual stimulation of the vagus nerve to slow the heart rate.

vagus nerve: The 10th cranial nerve, part of the parasympathetic nervous system. When stimulated, it slows the heart rate.

Valsalva's maneuver: Bearing down, or forced exhalation effort against a closed glottis, which slows the heart rate.

Wolff-Parkinson-White syndrome: A disorder characterized by accelerated atrioventricular conduction, producing rapid heart rates.

Selected References

Abels, Linda F. *Mosby's Manual of Critical Care: Practices and Procedures, Ninteen Seventy-Nine.* St. Louis: C.V. Mosby Co., 1979.

Andreoli, Kathleen, et al. *Comprehensive Cardiac Care,* 4th ed. St. Louis: C.V. Mosby Co., 1979.

Benchimol, Alberto. *Non-Invasive Techniques in Cardiology.* Baltimore: Williams & Wilkins Co., 1977.

Berne, Robert M., and Levy, Matthew N. *Cardiovascular Physiology,* 3rd ed. St. Louis: C.V. Mosby Co., 1977.

Boscala, M., et al. *Clinical Elements of Fetal Heart Rate Monitoring.* Waltham, Mass.: Hewlett-Packard, 1977.

Brehm, J.J., et al. *The Heart, Arteries, and Veins.* New York: McGraw-Hill Book Co., 1978.

Brunner, Lillian S. *The Lippincott Manual of Nursing Practice,* 2nd ed. Philadelphia: J.B. Lippincott Co., 1978.

Brunner, Lillian S., et al. *Textbook of Medical-Surgical Nursing,* 4th ed. Philadelphia: J.B. Lippincott Co., 1980.

Burrell, Zeb, Jr., and Burrell, Lennette O. *Critical Care,* 3rd ed. St. Louis: C.V. Mosby Co., 1977.

Disch, Joann M. *Diagnostic Procedures for Cardiovascular Disease.* New York: Appleton-Century-Crofts, 1979.

Drugs, 2nd ed. Nurse's Reference Library, Springhouse, Pa.: Springhouse Corporation, 1984.

Ensuring Intensive Care. Nursing Photobook Series. Springhouse, Pa.: Springhouse Corporation, 1981.

Fink, Burton W. *Congenital Heart Disease: A deductive Approach to its Diagnosis.* Chicago: Year Book Medical Publishers, Inc., 1975.

Furman, Seymour. "Recent Developments in Cardiac Pacing," *Heart & Lung.* 7:813-826, September/October 1978.

Giving Cardiac Care. Nursing Photobook Series. Springhouse, Pa.: Springhouse Corporation, 1981.

Hill, D.W. and Dolan, A.M. *Instrumentation for Intensive Care.* New York: Grune & Stratton, 1976.

Hudak, Carolyn M. *Critical Care Nursing,* 2nd ed. Philadelphia: J.B. Lippincott Co., 1977.

Hurst, J. Willis. *The Heart.* New York: McGraw-Hill Book Co., 1978.

McKinney, B. *Pathology of the Cardiomyopathies.* Woburn, Mass.: Butterworth Publishers, Inc., 1977.

Meltzer, Lawrence E., et al. *Intensive Coronary Care: A Manual for Nurses,* 3rd ed. Bowie, Md.: Charles Press Publishers, 1977.

Miller, S., et al. *Methods in Critical Care—the A.A.C.N. Manual.* Philadelphia: W.B. Saunders Co., 1980.

Perloff, Joseph K. *The Clinical Recognition of Congenital Heart Disease,* 2nd ed. Philadelphia: W.B. Saunders Co., 1978.

Using Monitors. Nursing Photobook Series. Springhouse, Pa.: Springhouse Corporation, 1980.

Wilson, Robert Francis, ed. *Principles and Techniques of Critical Care.* Kalamazoo, Mich.: Upjohn Co., 1976.

Index